Martha McLaughlin has filled a much-needed niche in the literary world with her book, *Chemicals and Christians: Compassion and Caution.* This incredible resource is packed with practical information, helpful strategies, and numerous websites for both the novice and those experienced in dealing with chemical sensitivities. My husband has been suffering with chemical illness for over twenty-five years, and I heartily applaud her vision for encouraging churches and individuals to "see the unintended effects of products we use and to see the almost invisible and largely unreached people group of the chemically sensitive." Church boards everywhere should have at least one leader read this and be versed in helping their churches make safer decisions for their congregations.

Throughout the book, Martha gives the reader a firsthand look into the lives of tens, if not hundreds of people affected by chemical sensitivities. She expertly weaves together their heart-wrenching but very real stories with practical action tips for the chemically ill as well as for churches and individuals who are not yet affected. Her years of experience and connection with the chemical illness community, along with thorough research, show through on every page (including an appendix full of documentation and numerous resources). Look for spiritual as well as physical helps and insights and an emphasis on being proactive while also offering help for those who already suffer.

—Merry Marinello,
Author of *Invisible Illness, Visible God*

In this thought-provoking book, Martha does a fantastic job bringing to light and explaining the issue of chemical sensitivity. She gives practical tips for consumers on how they can be proactive in preventing health challenges related to toxic chemical exposures. Additionally, this book serves as a great resource for churches, educating them on how they can provide a "safer" environment for their congregations. Both ministry leaders and lay people will benefit greatly from this book.

—Janine Ridings
Founder/Director of Aroma of Christ Ministry
Author of *Comfort in the Storm*

Chemicals and Christians is the most comprehensive book on Multiple Chemical Sensitivity that I have ever found. This book covers everything from physical aspects to emotional and relationship concerns to spiritual encouragement. Martha has done a tremendous amount of research, and each chapter has a long list of footnotes. Every chapter also includes numerous, very helpful "Take Care" tips and great discussion questions. The resource section at the end contains over one hundred resources/links!

Martha shares the stark truth without pulling any punches but also with a grace that leaves one feeling encouraged. The book deals with many serious topics, but I came away optimistic for change, validated in my experiences, and comforted that I am not "the only one."

For those with MCS, Martha includes many ideas on how to cope and thrive despite the almost insurmountable odds. For those supporting someone with MCS, she helps the reader see what it feels like to have MCS. She shares many quotes from people who have been through this. For those who have barely heard of MCS, Martha helps explain what MCS is and why everyone in our world should care about it. Chemicals affect everyone, not just those with MCS.

Dr. Grace Ziem's lovely foreword in the book gives excellent perspective on the premise of the book, not to mention a physician's "weight" to what Martha has written.

Do yourself and your fellow human beings a favor and read this book!

—Christa Upton
Author of *MCS: Banished from the Human Race* and
*Building a House for Multiple Chemical Sensitivity:
A Mold-Resistant, Low-Tox Home*

—————⬦—————

"Out of sight, out of mind," for many of us, might be an appropriate description of chemicals that induce illness. Such compounds are typically invisible and ignored by most, yet they permeate countless items in our contemporary world. The possibility that everyday products might make people sick is an uncomfortable topic that many people would prefer to leave out of sight, out of mind. Individuals trying to avoid the substances that make them sick often need to isolate themselves from their surrounding chemical-laden communities, so they too become out of sight, out of mind. Martha McLaughlin, in her book *Chemicals and Christians* urges the Christian family of faith to open our eyes to see and take action to care about the people with chemical sensitivities whom we have excluded from our fellowship by our lack of awareness, casual indifference, and impoverished hospitality.

Bringing the invisible into both sight and mind, *Chemicals and Christians* guides readers through the disturbing stages commonly experienced by persons who find their lives devastated by health problems that they eventually trace to exposure to synthetic chemicals. Such chemicals, pervasive in our modern world, are as common as fragrances and fabric softeners. Those most affected by chemical illness may regain a level of health by avoiding social situations fraught with chemical hazards. Yet the cost is severe isolation, including exclusion from their faith communities. Christian congregations would do well to examine how our practices are unintentionally barring persons with chemically induced illness from entering and participating. Not an easy book to read, *Chemicals and Christians* nevertheless offers an important call to faith communities to repent of toxic and inhospitable habits, so that vulnerable people whom Christ loves might find safety and hospitality in our midst and we all might find wholeness.

—Christine Guth
Retired Program Director
Anabaptist Disabilities Network

Chemicals and Christians confirms what I have already learned from living with an MCS afflicted wife. We couldn't understand what was happening to her health until we began connecting her symptoms to her exposure to one chemical after another. Our eyes have been opened to so many unnecessary chemicals that have become a part of life today.

Martha McLaughlin highlights many of these "unnecessary" chemicals, chemicals we can do without if we would only open our eyes to the danger they are to our good health. She has done a remarkable job of assimilating stories of individuals and their families living with MCS. Some will read this book and "learn" while others will read it and "scoff" until it is too late for them and they join the ranks of MCS sufferers. Thank you, Martha, for this exposure of the danger of "chemical overload" to our bodies and our good health. God bless you!

—Rev. Marcus Kuehn

In *Chemicals and Christians* Martha McLaughlin effectively makes the case that everyone, both the still-healthy and the sick, should be concerned about exposures to chemicals and learn how to protect themselves. At least 11 percent of the population suffers from diagnosed multiple chemical sensitivity (MCS), and many more are not diagnosed or have chemically-caused illnesses that are not recognized as MCS. Government regulations are woefully inadequate for protection, labels can be misleading, and the medical profession commonly misdiagnoses MCS and can do more harm than good. The incidence of MCS has been rising. Therefore, we all need the information in this book to restore or preserve our health.

For those already sick, she tells how to sift through our environments, discover what products and materials in our homes, churches, workplaces, and schools are causing symptoms, and how to avoid toxic exposures. She also discusses making wise decisions about potential treatments; how to resolve problems with finding safe food, clothing, and shelter; emotional, relational and spiritual needs; and the grief-anger issues experienced with MCS. Especially helpful and unique to this book are the sections on relationships with others, a balanced biblical perspective on healing, and the rediscovery of gratitude, purpose and that God is all we need. An extensive resources section is included to aid those with MCS in finding products, services, and sources of support and information they need.

Martha speaks from years of personal experience and much research in both medical sources and the Bible. Every Christian with MCS or who has a family member or friend with MCS needs this book. Every church needs it to effectively minister to chemically sensitive members of the body of Christ.

—Nicolette Dumke
Author of *Healing Basics* and
The Low Dose Immunotherapy Handbook
http://healingbasics.life

CHEMICALS
— *and* —
CHRISTIANS

*Compassion
and Caution*

MARTHA McLAUGHLIN

CHEMICALS
—— and ——
CHRISTIANS

*Compassion
and Caution*

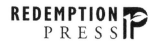
REDEMPTION
PRESS

© 2020 by Martha McLaughlin. All rights reserved.

Published by Redemption Press, PO Box 427, Enumclaw, WA 98022.

Toll-Free (844) 2REDEEM (273-3336)

Redemption Press is honored to present this title in partnership with the author. The views expressed or implied in this work are those of the author. Redemption Press provides our imprint seal representing design excellence, creative content, and high-quality production.

No part of this publication may be reproduced, stored in a retrieval system, or transmitted in any way by any means—electronic, mechanical, photocopy, recording, or otherwise—without the prior permission of the copyright holder, except as provided by USA copyright law.

The author has tried to recreate events, locales, and conversations from her memories of them. In order to maintain their anonymity, in some instances she has changed the names of individuals and may have changed some identifying characteristics and details, such as physical properties, occupations, and places of residence.

Unless otherwise indicated, all Scripture quotations are taken from the Holy Bible, New Living Translation, copyright © 1996, 2004, 2015 by Tyndale House Foundation. Used by permission of Tyndale House Publishers, Inc., Carol Stream, Illinois 60188. All rights reserved.

Scripture quotations marked CEV are taken from the Contemporary English Version Copyright © 1991, 1992, 1995 by American Bible Society. Used by permission.

Scripture quotations marked NIV are from THE HOLY BIBLE, NEW INTERNATIONAL VERSION®, NIV® Copyright © 1973, 1978, 1984, 2011 by Biblica, Inc.® Used by permission. All rights reserved worldwide.

Scripture quotations marked HCSB are taken from the Holman Christian Standard Bible®, Copyright © 1999, 2000, 2002, 2003, 2009 by Holman Bible Publishers. Used by permission. Holman Christian Standard Bible®, Holman CSB®, and HCSB® are federally registered trademarks of Holman Bible Publishers.

All Scripture marked MSG taken from The Message. Copyright © 1993, 1994, 1995, 1996, 2000, 2001, 2002. Used by permission of NavPress Publishing Group.

All Scripture quotations marked KJV taken from the King James Version, which is public domain.

Editing by Linda Nathan, Logos Word Designs, LLC (http://www.logosword.com)

ISBN: 978-1-68314-896-8 (paperback)
          978-1-68314-897 (epub)
          978-1-68314-898-2 (mobi)

Library of Congress Catalog Card Number: 2019934497

CONTENTS

FOREWORD 1

INTRODUCTION 5

CHAPTER ONE: Sicken 9
What Are the Common Symptoms of Chemical Illness? 11
How Does Someone Develop the Condition? 17
How Many People Are Affected? 22
What Chemicals Are Usually Implicated? 27
Doesn't the Government Protect Us? 33

CHAPTER TWO: Search 37
Diagnosis Prognosis 37
Stress and Distress 40
The Moment of Discovery 50

CHAPTER THREE: Sift 53
Forgoing Fragrance 54
Healthy Homes 57

CHAPTER FOUR: Separate 73
Community Concerns 73
The Working World 75
Learning Lessons 79
Shopping Shocks 82
Doctoring Dangers 85
The Trouble with Travel 86
The Move to Masks 91
The Challenge of Church 96

CHAPTER FIVE: Strike 103
Unlimited Options; Limited Funds 103
To Doctor or Not to Doctor 107
Decisions, Decisions 110

CHAPTER SIX: Sigh 119
   Physical Needs 120
   Emotional Needs 129
   Spiritual Needs 139

CHAPTER SEVEN: Scream 147
   Labeled 147
   Blamed 150
   Viewed as a Problem 152
   Beaten with the Bible 154
   Judged like Job 161
   Pummeled with Prayer 165
   Disappointed in the Divine 168

CHAPTER EIGHT: Seethe 173
   Indignant at Indifference 173
   Fighting Goliath 179
   Screaming into the Wind 187
   Taking Sides 189

CHAPTER NINE: Salvage 193
   Body 193
   Soul 194
   Spirit 202

CHAPTER TEN: Smile 215
   Awareness Activities 215
   Freedom from Fragrance 217
   Safer Schools 218
   Healthier Healthcare 220
   Progress with Pesticides 221
   Church Changes 222

RESOURCES 231
   Christian Health-Related Ministries 231
   Christian Chemical Illness Support Groups 232
   Church-Related Articles and Information Pages 233
   Christian Teaching and Bible Study Tools 234
   General Chemical Illness and Toxin Awareness Resources ... 234

Product Safety Information 236
Healthy Building and Renovation 237
Safer Housing 239
Nontoxic Cleaning 240
Lawn Care and Pest Management 240
Personal Care Products 242
Travel 242
Workplace Accommodation 242
Healthcare 243
Safer Schools 244

DISCUSSION QUESTIONS 245

CHURCH CHECKLIST 251

ENDNOTES 255

FOREWORD

Chemicals and Christians makes an important contribution to all of us because we all live in an increasingly chemicalized environment. I specialize in caring for patients whose lives have been permanently harmed by chemical exposure, which has limited their ability to be safe at home with their neighbors' use of chemicals, to utilize schools, and to work. They often have serious difficulty obtaining reasonable accommodations on the job even if they can become healthy enough to return to employment.

This book offers a very significant contribution by relating the experiences of toxic victims and their vital need for spiritual support. When churches understand the need for accommodation, they are more likely than the typical employer to provide it because of the Christian values of loving others as we love ourselves and as Christ loves us.

If Christians understand and follow the teachings of Christ, they can provide kindness, love, and support to those trying to navigate the chemicalized world, who frequently are lonely and endure rude treatment by those who do not understand or who do not want to be bothered. Other church members will benefit from reducing their own use of toxic products such as petroleum-based scented products (that are not made from flowers these days), fabric softener (which creates a respiratory particulate that clings to clothing and is scattered throughout the house, car, and every environment that a person enters), and pesticide residues.

Churches and others can benefit from knowing that there are nontoxic alternatives for all of these situations. Pests can be controlled through nontoxic methods. The 501(c)(3) organization Beyond Pesticides has an excellent science-based website: beyondpesticides.org. They discuss the toxicity of various pesticides and effective nontoxic alternatives. The use of fabric softener can often be avoided by using less detergent (about a fourth or less of the manufacturer's "recommended" amount effectively cleans and leaves less residue to be "softened"). For people living in areas where the water is hard, a water softener is a much safer approach, and it will save medical bills.

I have been practicing medicine for forty-five years. During that time I have seen a dramatic increase of autoimmune disease, "allergies," attention deficit and hyperactivity, chronic fatigue, widespread aching/"fibromyalgia," neurodegenerative diseases, and cancer. People may be unaware that cardiovascular disease and diabetes are also now known to be diseases of chronic inflammation. These illnesses share significant overlapping of biochemical disturbance with chemical illness, but they have no earlier warning system such as headaches or respiratory irritation to protect and warn people that their environments are too toxic for their bodies. Because the introduction of chemicals into the environment has dramatically increased in the last three to four decades, and we have a dramatic increase of chronic inflammatory diseases, as mentioned above, we all need to pay serious attention to what is happening to the precious planet that God gave us.

These exposures were not present in the days when the Bible was written. However, readers may be interested in the discussion in Leviticus relating to mold. This is an advanced approach that I consider to be God's founding of the first school of public health. In addition to outlining preventive measures for other illnesses, Leviticus (14:37–53) warns the Israelites and readers that if they see visible mold in a dwelling, they should remove all mold-contaminated substances. There should be a subsequent reinspection. If there is a recurrence of the mold, God instructs people to remove the entire dwelling and carry it outside of the town for proper disposal. Thus, over three thousand years ago, God gave us an excellent mold remediation program, which has yet to be implemented. This approach to mold would have prevented the mold-induced illness that I see in my practice. The general focus of the precautions in Leviticus is that the problem should be removed and safer products used. I completely agree.

Using safe approaches regarding chemicals is not only Christian, but is also good sense. A bird will change its nest each year. However, we apply a new carpet, fresh paint, fabric softener, plastic toys, and other products to the nurseries of our precious babies and children. We then wonder why they have so much respiratory irritation, as well as so many learning disabilities, behavioral changes, and so forth. When are we going to get the message our children are trying to give us? When are we going to stop poisoning the planet our Lord has provided for us? When are we going to pay serious attention to persons who have difficulty with our pattern of chemical use, and thank them for pointing out a serious problem that affects us all? Do we want to spend our last days on this planet with chronic inflammatory disease or neurodegenerative disease in a long-term care facility, or would we like to be healthy in our older years? God has given us this choice. Let us choose to protect ourselves, our children, and our planet.

—————•◆•—————

Dr. Ziem specializes in the prevention and treatment of chemically related illness. She has, in addition to her MD degree, a master of public health from Johns Hopkins, and a master of science and a doctor of public health from Harvard.

INTRODUCTION

M ost people living today would probably agree that chemicals can make us sick. We may have a tendency, though, to think of "chemicals" in vague and distant terms—as manufacturing spills or toxic emissions we might hear about in the news. "Sick," in this way of thinking, usually seems to mean developing cancer or another disease we can easily tie to the problematic products. It happens to unfortunate others, we're tempted to think, and has limited relevance to us.

Industrial waste is a major concern, and chemical exposures are definitely tied to cancers and a wide range of known diseases. The challenges posed by modern chemicals, however, are much broader and deeper than our culture and our churches seem to realize. The truth is that all of us marinate daily in a broth of synthetic, man-made products that in ordinary amounts can have serious effects on our bodies, minds, and spirits. Because most of us aren't tuned to look for a connection or don't have the information we need about the products that surround us, we may be unaware that we're suffering the effects of chemical exposures.

Some people, however, have come to see a direct relationship between exposure to specific chemicals and the health symptoms they face. Although chemical exposure can worsen any health disorder, those who have significant and direct problems have a condition described by many names. These include environmental illness (EI), toxic illness, toxicant-induced loss of tolerance (TILT), chemical illness, chemical injury, multiple chemical sensitivity (MCS), and more.

This book discusses the chemicals found in common products. It's written for those who react to those chemicals, both knowingly and unknowingly, those whose actions affect people who are chemically ill, and those at risk of developing toxic illness. The categories include every human on earth. A key theme is that seemingly small decisions about the use of common products may affect people's wellbeing and that of those around them in profound and life-altering ways. Everyday items can make healthy people sick and sick people sicker.

To a large degree, this book is about the church and how it can help and harm people at all stages of chemical tolerance or reactivity. The message is simple: there's a large but seemingly invisible group of people who are currently not only unreached, but actually shut out of corporate fellowship. They need to be seen, not only for the sake of ministering to them, but for the warning they provide to others, who can very easily join their ranks.

The message in two words is this: take care. Take care not to let everyday chemicals affect you, and take care of those who've already developed toxic illness. This book will include "Take Care" Tips designed to help stimulate thinking along those lines and serve as a springboard for prayer and further ideas.

No one reading this book is immune to the effects of the toxins that fill our air, our food, our water, and our bodies. As a culture, we've been deceived into thinking we need products that are actually harming us. When the extent of the problem is understood, it may seem overwhelming or impossible to address, but no step forward is wasted. Some changes are actually fairly easy to make and can make a bigger difference to the health and wellbeing of the body of Christ than we might imagine. One step can lead to others. Education and motivation are the places to start, and my hope is that pulling back the curtain on the invisible world of toxic illness will help in that process.

I write this book as someone with connections both to the world of the chemically ill and to the Christian community. I was born into a pastor's family, came to know and love Jesus at an early age, attended a Christian college, and married a worship minister. We served as missionaries in South

America for ten years, but eventually my health no longer allowed me to serve overseas.

When I realized I could manage my symptoms by managing my exposure to chemicals, I found myself in a new world I hadn't known existed. As a missionary, I gave a lot of thought to "unreached people groups," but when I became ill, I suddenly found myself in a sense a part of one. My desire is for more of the Christian community to be aware of this world and to both learn from those reactive to chemicals and to take steps to reach out to them with the love of Christ.

I've been writing this book for a very long time. It was 99 percent complete when my husband suddenly died and my life, by necessity, became focused on other things. I return to it now with a sense of sadness that things have improved so little in the intervening years. Sometimes I see progress, sometimes I see regress, but mostly I see a huge need for Christians to become educated and to take the lead on this issue.

For the sake of organization, I've divided this book into chapters related to the stages of chemical illness I've identified in myself and others. These are loosely defined stages people can pass through in different orders and remain in for varying lengths of time. It's possible to identify with several stages at once or to return to a previous stage at any point. Some parts of this book will relate more directly to currently healthy people, and some to those who are ill, but I hope readers will engage with the entire message. We have much to learn from each other, and we're all in this together as we face the deception and lack of information that keep us from being aware of the chemical challenges around us.

Many chemically reactive individuals share their stories here. All are real people who've given permission for me to share their words, but in most cases, names have been changed to protect privacy and to allow for free expression of the frustration that's part of having toxic illness in our chemical-soaked society. The world of the chemically injured may seem strange to those who are healthy and not associated with the toxic illness community, but it's a real world, and we invite you in through this book. We truly desire for you to learn some things sooner than we did and in a less painful way. We also need your help. Thank you for taking the time to focus on the issue.

Nothing in this book should be considered medical advice.

CHAPTER ONE

Sicken

Intelligent people are always ready to learn.
Their ears are open for knowledge.
—Proverbs 18:15

When the alarm shattered the silence on Sunday morning, Mary sighed and pushed the "off" button groggily. She hadn't slept well. In fact, that was becoming a pattern lately. She perched on the side of her mattress, made of synthetic materials and treated with fire retardant, until she felt ready to stand and face the day. She hastily pulled up the wrinkle-resistant sheet and acrylic blanket and threw the comforter on top, which was likewise made of man-made fibers.

Mary began to prepare for church using synthetically fragranced and chemically derived body wash, shampoo, conditioner, and deodorant, then dressed in clothes she had washed in fragranced detergent and dried with chemical-laden dryer sheets. She decided to take an aspirin to stave off the slight headache she was feeling. Passing by the mirror made her frown. She had been slowly gaining weight and didn't appreciate the extra pounds.

There was only time for a quick breakfast, so Mary heated up some specialty tea in the microwave. The chemicals used to create the artificial fruit flavor filled the kitchen. She then set out cereal, which likewise contained artificial flavors and colors, for her family to grab. She could hear her children bickering in the other room. She loved her kids, but they sure were driving her crazy lately. They had so much energy, but they seemed unable to focus on anything she said to them and were constantly sick with colds or the flu.

By the time everyone made it to church, nerves were a bit on edge. The family walked by the weed-treated and chemically fertilized church lawn and entered the carpeted and well-decorated foyer, recently cleaned with heavily fragranced petroleum-based cleaners. When family members scattered and went their separate ways, Mary decided to swing by the church kitchen, floored in vinyl and equipped with particleboard cabinets and a gas stove, for a doughnut and cup of coffee. She was feeling a little foggy-headed.

Mary next headed to the classroom where her Bible study was held and noticed again how nice the recently painted walls looked. The teacher pulled out a dry erase marker to note prayer requests on the board, and, as usual, soon filled it with names of church members battling cancer and other serious health conditions. Mary noticed that numbers had been down in the class for the past few weeks. She wondered if some sort of bug was going around. She was just getting over a bout of bronchitis herself.

After the Bible study ended, Mary found her usual spot in the church sanctuary. A fellow member wearing cologne took a seat behind her. Mary didn't like the music today. The sermon wasn't very good either. In fact, she felt quite irritable in general. Mary evidently wasn't the only member not into the sermon this week. She looked around and could see a number of people who seemed to be struggling to stay awake.

Chemicals in the environment were affecting Mary and her fellow church members, and will continue to affect them. Some sitting in the pews with Mary will go through life and never suffer more than mild health problems. Some, however, will suffer from serious medical conditions related to chemical exposures, though they won't associate them. Others will eventually make the connection between chemical exposures and their health and will face the task of trying to stay well in a world that makes that very challenging.

———————

Every journey has a beginning, and the *Sicken* phase holds the starting gate for the demanding journey of toxic illness. In this phase, symptoms related to chemical exposures emerge and grow. How they begin varies among sufferers.

The onset of the illness can be either sudden and immediate or so gradual that at first it's barely noticed. Dr. Pamela Gibson surveyed sufferers and found that approximately 20 percent believed that one large exposure to a dangerous product caused their condition. More often though, respondents thought that a series of low-level exposures initiated the problem, with 59 percent putting themselves in that category. Other respondents blamed a physical illness (5%), a psychological stressor (less than 1%), said they didn't know (9%), or didn't answer the question (7%).[1]

It's very common for symptoms of chemical illness to sneak up gradually and for people to consider them insignificant at first. After all, who doesn't have a headache now and then, experience cold or flu-like symptoms, or develop fatigue, explainable by a hectic schedule? People in the *Sicken* stage tend to take over-the-counter medication and do their best to carry on daily activities without interruption.

Our world is full of people in the *Sicken* stage. Chemicals in the home, church, school, and work environments are affecting them, but they have no idea that a connection may exist between their symptoms and the products they and others use. If people in this stage have continued exposure to problematic chemicals, new health problems tend to arise or old problems become more intrusive. Symptoms may increase in frequency or intensity until they begin to interfere with daily life.

What Are the Common Symptoms of Chemical Illness?

No two people with toxic illness are exactly alike because specific toxins interact with individual biology in personal ways. Symptoms may have a variety of chemical-related causes, including irritant-induced inflammation, toxic encephalopathy (chemical damage to the brain), or neural sensitization (increased reactivity of the nervous system to stimuli). Dr. Nicolas Ashford provides the analogy of tossing magnets inside ten computers then asking each of them to add two plus two and getting different wrong answers from each. He says, "When you throw a neurotoxic chemical into the brain, and you know a lot of them get into the brain, including the limbic system, which is where the immune system, the nervous system, and endocrine system converge, they may make the brain misbehave in a number of different ways."[2]

Symptoms experienced in the early stages of chemical injury may differ from those experienced later. Prominent environmental health physician Dr. Grace Ziem notes that early warnings of chemical injury may involve the following symptoms:

- Irritation of eyes, nose, throat, and lungs
- Sinus headaches and migraines
- Poor memory and concentration
- Hyperactivity (especially in children)

Later, chemical injury may manifest itself in other ways such as the following:

- Chronic fatigue
- Widespread aching
- Autoimmune and degenerative diseases
- Cancer[3]

Personal physical differences affect symptomology. Ziem notes that children, for example, are more likely than adults to suffer from exposure-related earaches because of their small eustachian tubes.[4]

Chemical exposures can directly or indirectly affect every organ system. Following is a sampling of some of the diverse symptoms those with toxic illness may face as described by those who experience them:

> I don't think I really understood the meaning of the word tired until I got MCS and chemical reactions. I bet there are people of ninety who have more energy at those times.

I get fatigue and intestinal stuff a lot, but for me the worst symptom is the horrible muscle and nerve pain. It's truly, truly awful. I just lie on the bed and pray that God will help me get through one more day. Actually, sometimes I pray that I won't make it through one more day.

———✦———

I can unequivocally tell you that I definitely get itching and hives from exposure, and perfume is a biggy. I have hives tonight.

———✦———

I cried for three days once when staying with my daughter. Yes, I was under stress, but I don't usually cry. On the way home from her house, the crying stopped. It seems my son-in-law had used flakeboard in their downstairs shelving area, and the formaldehyde did me in. I couldn't smell it, but it sure did a number on me.

———✦———

Some of the ways the illness frustrates me are: weak muscles; deep coughing; pain in joints, muscles, back, and head; brain fog; low energy; overwhelming fatigue; inability to listen, speak, or interact much; insomnia; heart palpitations and anxiety; and inability to sort, make decisions, and organize.

———✦———

When I was still working, I knew that new carpeting bothered me but I didn't know why—just that I would get a
horrible cold when I was around new carpeting.

———————————————————

Certain chemicals make me stop sleeping. I can go for
weeks after an exposure where I barely sleep at all—maybe
an hour or two a night.

———————————————————

It took fifteen years of having to leave the sanctuary at
church for me to connect my coughing with printer's ink.
The coughing started a couple of minutes after everyone
opened their hymnals. It took longer than that to figure out
why I'd get a major migraine about three hours after exposures. That delayed reaction was SO strong, but it didn't
start until several hours later.

In"toxic"ation. At times, the effects of toxic chemicals can mimic being
drunk, high, or hungover. It isn't a coincidence that the word "intoxicat-
ed" contains a reference to the word "toxin." The practice and dangers of
"huffing" (deliberately inhaling the fumes from household products in an
attempt to get high) can also teach us about the effects of certain classes of
chemicals. The body doesn't care if the person inhales the fumes voluntarily
or involuntarily. The physical results are the same.

The National Institute on Drug Abuse notes the following among the
long list of possible effects of inhalants:

- Nausea
- Confusion
- Agitation
- Drowsiness

- Dizziness
- Muscle weakness
- Headaches[5]

Compare that list to further descriptions chemical illness sufferers give of their experiences.

> Usually I will get nausea the next day after leaving the house, but this time I got it within five hours. It's like those tsunami waves over, over, and over. I'm going to go lie down and hang onto a cat.

> The year before I quit my long-term employment was so interesting—bleeding in eye, lots of antibiotics, nausea from hell. I just had too many chemicals in my system. One of my coworkers was stressed out because I kept losing my purse. It didn't bother me as much as it did her. Most of the time I would get to work without my purse. One time I left my wallet lying on the front seat of my car with the doors unlocked. God was sure watching over my car as I found the wallet the next day when I got ready to go to work.

> Perfume makes me want to kill someone. I think I read that it has something to do with the limbic system. All I know is that it's a really intense rage that sometimes takes a huge amount of effort to control.

> I get dizzy, shaky, disoriented, lost (like Alzheimer's), headaches, forgetful, a speech impediment, a hearing impediment, my vision worsens, my appetite center stops working, I get cold, tired, cranky, I stress out more easily,

get angry or cry more easily, and my heartbeat changes. I lose my ability to spell and to comprehend or retain what I read. I lose my ability to use logic. I lose my ability to see patterns. I don't see colors correctly. I can't concentrate. I become really uncoordinated (bumping into things, unable to pick up a spoon without focusing on the action, tripping over my own toes).

When I'm exposed, I forget my phone number. That's normal for some people, but I have had the same phone number for thirty-five years.

Take Care Tip

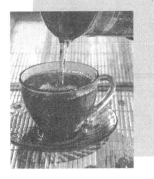

- If you or someone you love is suffering from unexplained health problems, consider keeping a journal or otherwise attempting to discern patterns that might show correlations with environmental exposures. If patterns aren't obvious, don't assume no chemical connection exists. Sometimes they're hard to see because of too many variables, but sometimes they're obvious once you think to look for them.

How Does Someone Develop the Condition?

Dr. Ziem describes the development of toxic illness this way:

> The types of substances that can initially cause toxic illness include solvents, combustion products, glues and adhesives, pesticides and herbicides and their residue, mold (because mold releases substances called "VOCs"), and the complex mixture of chemicals often found in building renovations. Many people are initially injured in an occupational setting because they are less able to control their environment or leave a problem area. Exposures in apartments and condominiums can also be a problem because people spend a lot of time in their homes. Some patients have a causal exposure in school, from pesticide misuse, poor ventilation, or chemicals used in vocational training and other programs.
>
> For most people, repeated exposures occur, each one causing symptoms, until the condition becomes chronic and can no longer be reversed to a healthy state. At this point, the body initiates a warning system to prevent further harmful exposure. Just like someone with a second-degree burn receives a strong body warning if they try to go out into bright sunlight, the body at some point of illness severity often develops a warning system. When this occurs, the person then experiences worsening of symptoms around exposure levels and durations that did not affect them when they were healthy. Their body produces warning symptoms that often relate to the areas that were initially harmed.[6]

Dr. Ziem stresses that the concept of an individual harmed by chemical or toxic exposure becoming more intolerant of further harm is not unique to chemicals, but rather a normal body defense mechanism. She points out that "someone with a sunburn is more sensitive to a 'pat on the back,' someone with an injured finger or hand is more intolerant of touch and motion involving the injured part, and someone with liver injury is more intolerant of medications and other substances that affect the liver. This applies to all organs. These are all ways God has designed our bodies to prevent further injury and thus help the healing process."[7]

Some try to paint chemical illness as a psychological disorder, an issue we'll discuss in subsequent chapters, but there's no shortage of research findings corroborating a physical, rather than a psychological, basis for the condition. A brief sampling of the research follows:

- Animal models point to a physical cause. Studies show that animals exposed to repeated low levels of chemicals over a period of time can become extremely reactive and sensitive to minute traces of those chemicals.[8]

- Researchers found that people who became sick after exposure to certain chemicals in Operation Desert Storm had lower amounts of a specific enzyme than did people who didn't get ill.[9]

- One study revealed that women with a genetic profile involving two genes associated with detoxifying toxic compounds were over eighteen times more likely to have MCS compared to women with a different genetic makeup. (I unfortunately have issues with these two genes myself.) Women with variations in just one of the implicated genes were also more likely to develop chemical sensitivities.[10]

- Researchers have found nasal abnormalities consistent with chronic inflammation in patients with chemical illness. Damaged mucosa enhances absorption of inhaled chemicals and often permits rapid entry into the brain.[11]

- Testing often shows people who react to chemicals are "pathological detoxifiers" in which Phase I of liver detoxification is faster than Phase II, which leads to a buildup of toxic metabolites in the body.

- Groups of independent researchers have found distinct abnormalities of brain metabolism in people with chemical illness. The neurotoxic pattern is very different from the abnormalities reported in psychiatric disease.[12]

- Tests measuring blood flow to the brain (SPECT scans) show differences between chemically sensitive patients and normal controls. Chemically reactive patients demonstrate severe deterioration when they're challenged by chemicals in concentrations found in everyday situations.[13]

In his book *12,000 Canaries Can't Be Wrong*, Dr. John Molot says:

> The sciences of genetics, cell biology, and chemical toxicology, supported by animal models and proper challenge studies in humans, attest to the fact that susceptible people can become sensitized to multiple different chemicals, with resulting illness and disability. . . . The weight of evidence is robust. . . . The statement, "There is no science to support the existence of MCS" now borders on ignorance.[14]

A self-perpetuating problem. Chemical illness can become a self-perpetuating problem because chemicals can damage the body's detoxification system, which leads to more difficulty processing toxins. Genetic differences exist in people's abilities to detoxify, but chemicals can affect even these, both mutating genes and affecting their expression. Some substances, such as heavy metals like lead and mercury, can affect the barrier that protects the brain and make it easier for other chemicals to enter.[15]

Some chemicals, known as sensitizers, are more likely to initiate toxic illness than others. Sensitizers may initially cause no discernible effects, but repeated exposures make people more likely to develop reactions, both to the original chemical and to others. One author explains that "seven classes of chemicals, including solvents and . . . pesticides, have the capacity to induce the vicious cycle now known to underlie MCS."[16]

Related health conditions. Chemical illness goes by many names and can contribute to and accompany many health conditions. Some believe that Gulf War Syndrome is, essentially, just another name for toxic illness. A National Academy of Sciences study reported on the link between Gulf

War Syndrome and chemical exposures.[17] Dr. Beatrice Golomb, the study's author, stated that "enough studies have been conducted . . . to be able to say with considerable confidence that there is a link between chemical exposure and chronic, multi-symptom health problems." Golomb added that "the same chemicals affecting Gulf War veterans may be involved in similar cases of unexplained, multi-symptom health problems in the general population."[18]

Chemical reactivity can be the body's way of saying, "I'm dealing with too much right now and don't have the resources to devote to detoxifying everything coming at me." People sometimes refer to the total load or "rain barrel" theory, which is the idea that our bodies have limited capacity for dealing with toxins, much as a rain barrel has a limited capacity for holding rain. If the level in our barrel is high, we can handle very little additional toxic exposure before becoming overwhelmed, but if our level is low, we can handle significantly more.

Many things can contribute to raising our load. Chemical toxins contribute, of course, but so do nonchemical stressors like viral or bacterial infections and mold exposure. In my own case, my genetically weak detoxification system became overwhelmed not just by man-made toxins but by mold exposure and Lyme disease.

Food reactions are a common accompaniment to chemical illness. Sometimes actual food allergies or intolerances cause the symptoms and sometimes chemicals do. Fruits and vegetables may have pesticide residue, and meats may contain hormones or antibiotics. Artificial and even so-called "natural" flavors added to food products often contain scores of chemical compounds. Eric Schlosser, author of the book *Fast Food Nation,* explains that artificial and natural flavorings often contain the same mixture of chemicals, simply produced through different methods. He notes that the world's largest flavor company manufactures the fragrances of six of the ten best-selling American perfumes and those found in many household cleaning and personal care products. He says, "All these aromas are made through essentially the same process: the manipulation of volatile chemicals. The basic science behind the scent of your shaving cream is the same as that governing the flavor of your TV dinner."[19]

Canaries and miners. The simplest explanation for chemical illness is that toxic chemicals have toxic effects. Lynn Lawson, in her book *Staying*

Well in a Toxic World, quotes someone who puts it this way. "If your kid plays in the street and is run over by a truck, do you say, 'Poor thing, he's sensitive to Fords?' We're basically dealing with poisons, not frail health."[20]

The chemically reactive often call themselves canaries, after the canaries that coal miners once took with them into the mines. Because canaries were more sensitive to the mine gas than their human partners, it would affect them first and warn the miners of danger. If the miners ignored the warning, the gas would affect them, too, sometimes fatally. The chemicals in our environment can overcome anyone. Some of us just show the effects more quickly or in ways that produce noticeable symptoms instead of more silent damage.

Dr. Mark Donohoe, in his book *Killing Us Softly*, writes:

> Let us reverse totally the view of MCS. MCS is neither an illness nor a disease. It is entirely normal. Not having MCS, however, is a real problem. What if the environment were incompatible with normal, healthy life? And what if this environment arose over a single generation or so? What would a successful biological response to this threat look like? . . . The biologically successful response would be one which could identify and minimize such exposure. One which could induce a sufficiently strong aversion response to prevent ongoing risk and damage. MCS. MCS sufferers may not be "broken" but the environment which induces an MCS response may well be bad for health. . . . MCS may, in short, be an adaptation to a lousy environment by developing the skills to avoid such environmental exposure. Those with MCS may, in fact, be the most normal people in the world. One could even suggest they are advanced compared to the rest of us, with a heightened sense able to detect and minimize risk for survival.[21]

Attempting to fully understand the etiology of a disease is certainly a worthwhile endeavor. However, as Nicolas Ashford and Claudia Miller point out in their book *Chemical Exposures: Low Levels and High Stakes*, "knowing the mechanism of a disease is not necessary in order to prevent it." They tell of a nineteenth century London doctor who noticed that people developing cholera were obtaining their water from a specific pump. The doctor, John Snow, stopped the epidemic by having the pump handle removed, even though scientists didn't discover the cholera bacterium for another thirty years.[22] If we can determine a cause and effect relationship between a chemical exposure and a negative physical state, the prudent course of action is to remove the cause of the distress.

Take Care Tips

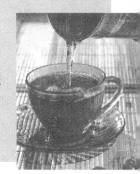

- Make it a goal to lower your toxic load in whatever way possible and to do your best not to sicken yourself or others.

- Begin to educate yourself about the toxicity of commonly used products. The resource list at the back of this book may prove helpful.

How Many People Are Affected?

An unavoidable and important fact is that the products in our environment are affecting all of us because any product in the environment will soon be in our bodies. The exposures start even before birth. Tests of umbilical cords show that a newborn's body contains nearly three hundred compounds.[23]

Changes both to the way genes are coded and the way they're expressed can have effects that are passed down for generations. Children in the womb can be affected by chemicals their mothers are exposed to, of course, but the issue goes far beyond that. Children can be affected by chemicals either of their parents has been exposed to even before the children are conceived. As one reporter notes, "Science reveals that the harmful effects of exposure to synthetic chemicals are passed from generation to generation via 'epigenetics,' causing measurable damage to future generations *even if those offspring are never exposed to the original chemical.*"[24] A World Health Organization publication states that "exposure of either mother or father to pesticides before conception . . . has been associated with an increased risk of fetal death, spontaneous abortion and early childhood cancer."[25]

The situation doesn't improve once we escape the womb. We can breathe chemicals in, swallow them, or our skin can absorb them. However they enter, enter they will. We are human sponges.

Untested chemicals surround us and fill us, but what percentage of the population is bothered by them to a significant and obvious extent? Although an exact number is hard to quantify, a safe response is, "a lot more than you might think." Researchers have conducted various studies. Some looked at specific populations such as young people, the elderly, or veterans, and found rates of chemical illness as high as a staggering 86 percent (among Gulf War veterans who were hospital outpatients).[26]

Studies of the general population have found rates that vary between 11 and 33 percent. The most recent study, involving more than one thousand adult Americans, found that 25.9 percent reported chemical sensitivity and 12.8 percent reported medically diagnosed MCS.

The Prevalence of Chemical Sensitivity			
Study Authors	Percentage of respondents unusually or especially sensitive to everyday chemicals	Percentage of respondents suffering daily or almost daily symptoms	Percentage of respondents officially diagnosed with MCS
Meggs, Dunn, and Bloch	33%	4%	
Voorhees	16%		2%
Kreutzer, Neutra, and Lashuay	16%		6%
Caress and Steinemann	11.2%		2.5%
Steinemann	25.9%		12.8%

(Note the following citations for the above authors: Meggs, Dunn, and Bloch[27]; Voorhees[28]; Kreutzer, Neutra, and Lashuay[29] Caress and Steinemann[30]; Steinemann.[31])

Evidently, somewhere between a tenth and a third of the population consider themselves unusually sensitive to chemical exposures and the number appears to be rising. Anne Steinmann, author of the most recent study, notes that "prevalence of diagnosed MCS has increased over 300 percent, and self-reported chemical sensitivity over 200 percent, in the past decade."[32]

Unaware, but not unaffected. The studies yield high numbers, but an important aspect of reported prevalence rates is that they only reflect people who *know* that chemicals cause their symptoms. They don't include those who have more silent illness or who aren't aware that their illness is chemically related. Undoubtedly, the number of people suffering the effects of chemicals without being aware of the connection is many magnitudes higher.

Part of the difficulty with making the connection is due to the sheer number of chemicals most people encounter. Alison Johnson, author of *Casualties of Progress*, a compilation of stories of the chemically sensitive, explains that "As [people] go through a day, symptoms triggered by fragrances, hair spray, vehicle exhaust, foods, and medications pile up so they feel sick most of the time. No one cause can be isolated because there's too much background noise."[33]

Obviously, lack of knowledge about chemical effects doesn't stop them from occurring. It just keeps people from protecting themselves. When people with health complaints are evaluated for chemical intolerance, it's generally found. Dr. Howard Kipen found that 54 percent of asthmatics met the threshold score for MCS on an exposure questionnaire, as did 20 percent of general medicine clinic patients.[34] A questionnaire given to 400 patients recruited from two family medicine clinics in Texas found a similar rate of 20.3 percent.[35]

People may also be unaware of the problems that common products are causing them because chemicals can cause much internal damage without immediately observable effects. Miller and Ashford explain that "acute symptoms gradually may give way to chronic symptoms that bear no apparent relationship to any particular exposure. Exposures may never stop long enough for the patient to reach baseline."[36] When people first begin smoking, for example, they may have immediate health effects (coughing), but if they continue to smoke, the coughing might disappear and be replaced with shortness of breath, chronic hoarseness, and more frequent colds. With or without observable symptoms, the risk for cancer and heart disease also increases. In the same way, those who don't immediately get a headache from perfume aren't immune to its health-damaging effects. Dr. Thomas Stone states that "the price we pay for chronic adaptation is chronic illness."[37]

Dr. Ziem notes:

> There has been a major increase in toxic-related conditions in the general population, such as autoimmune disease, attention deficit and/or hyperactivity, neurodegenerative diseases (Alzheimer's, Parkinson's, multiple sclerosis, and ALS), and numerous chronic inflammatory diseases. As more understanding becomes available about the bio-chemistry of these illnesses and the exposures of people who develop them, it is becoming increasingly evident that chemically-related illness is not limited to those who observe exacerbations, but could include millions of people who do not observe an exacerbation or do not have enough time with their physician to communicate the relationship.[38]

Sometimes a chemical connection to a health condition is "officially" known, but sufferers aren't generally aware of it. For example, the American Heart Association states that exposure to air pollution over a few hours to weeks can trigger cardiovascular disease, that longer-term exposure can reduce life expectancy by several months to a few years and that reductions in pollution levels are associated with reductions in cardiovascular deaths.[39] In my experience, however, it's rare for people to link their heart conditions to the air they breathe.

If a minimum of 11 percent of the population is very sensitive to the effects of common chemicals (the true rate is probably much, much higher), why isn't our society more aware of that? There are many facets to the answer, some of which involve special interests with deep pockets, and we'll discuss the topic later in this book. One simple truth is that the people most seriously affected by toxic illness are hidden away, avoiding chemical exposures as much as humanly possible, and as a result, they rarely participate in the cultural activities that would bring them into contact with the public.

There are a number of reasons those with toxic illness are sometimes hesitant to reveal their condition. Reactions to chemicals are not only poorly understood but often ridiculed, so people may learn that disclosing their condition can add emotional suffering to their physical symptoms and earn them a label as crazy or manipulative. People may also feel that talking about their reactions will offend or inconvenience others who may take requests to change their personal care products, for example, very personally, so they sometimes make the choice to pay a physical price to avoid that. Finally, some with chemical illness have learned that discussing their condition can give ill-intentioned people an easy way to cause them great harm.

How many is too many? The number of people seriously affected by common chemicals is an important question. Another is how many people must suffer before the not-yet-obviously-reactive make changes in order to protect themselves and those who share the air. It's time to face the issue. It's time to ask questions about the toxicity of our homes, schools, workplaces, and churches. It's time to seriously consider the ramifications of using the products we do, which may very well be sickening us and those around us too. God has entrusted us with an important responsibility. We're to care for the earth, for ourselves, and for the fellow pilgrims on this journey.

If someone were standing outside your church with an armful of packages, wanting to come in but needing help with the door, would you open it? If someone wanted to worship with you but needed an aisle seat because her leg was in a cast, would you provide the seat? What if someone desperately wanted to know more about Christ but needed you to provide clean air inside your building so he could hear the Word of God? Would you do that for him? What if that person were your son, your sister, your best friend, or your mother?

The changes that would allow the chemically ill to safely enter a church environment may also allow many currently healthy people to remain that way. Some changes are easy to make. Some are more challenging. Are they worth making? It's a question that deserves serious consideration.

Take Care Tip

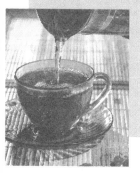

- Don't be afraid to tactfully discuss the issue of product toxicity and air quality in public spaces with those who share the air. You may be advocating for a larger group of people than you realize. Don't be surprised with either opposition or support. Either way, making indoor environments healthier for all is part of loving our neighbors as ourselves.[40]

WHAT CHEMICALS ARE USUALLY IMPLICATED?

Those who suffer obvious ill effects from low levels of chemical exposures have had difficulty settling on an appropriate name for the condition. One limitation of the designation "chemical sensitivity" is that "sensitivity" fails to communicate the intensity and seriousness of reactions suffered. The term "chemical" is also broad and amorphous, but there doesn't seem to be a better term to describe the products that initiate most symptoms.

Chemical triggers are everywhere. They can be in the form of vapors and gases or tiny particles too small to see. They may or may not have a noticeable odor. When chemicals are used, human exposure is likely, whether or not the chemicals are seen, smelled, or otherwise obvious.

Beth talks about some of the exposures that led to her chemical illness.

> They did a major remodel at work. I had a newer car. I lived across the street from a swimming pool (chlorine), lived upwind from a freeway, and had a stop sign right outside my patio and a parking lot outside my open bedroom window (car exhaust). I lived a short distance from a huge

community laundry room (detergents and fabric softeners). I got a large Christmas bonus, so I bought a new computer desk, had my carpet cleaned, got a new computer monitor and new clothes.

I had become very sensitive to the toner of the copiers at work. The maintenance man told me that the copiers needed to be vented, but they weren't. Then my employer installed four perfumed air fresheners in the bathrooms. That was the last straw for me. I could tell within five minutes that the air fresheners had been replaced. The owner of the building refused to remove them. I got worse until I was afraid that I was going to die.

Melissa's story is also typical.

I'm not sure exactly how long I've had MCS. I started working in the church office as a full-time secretary. I remember going into work feeling fine and then getting extremely tired and feeling like I was in a brain fog. I felt better in the evenings at home. Then I started having seizures. After I quit working there, the seizures stopped. Then I got married and had my children and remember getting really sick when we bought our house and the previous owner had it sprayed inside for a bad infestation of fleas. I didn't think much about it at the time and then very slowly started having occasional problems with very strong cleaning chemicals and secondhand cigarette smoke.

I had surgery and months of antibiotics and pain meds. I slowly started to recover and then realized I was having problems with allergies, asthma attacks, sinus infections, memory problems, digestion issues, etc.

I went back to work at my church as an assistant preschool teacher. After being there a short time, I started coming home sick every day. I slowly began to realize that the asthma and many other symptoms were coming from chemicals and perfumes. I still didn't know that MCS existed and kept going back and getting sicker.

Newly built or remodeled buildings are a common chemical illness or "sick building syndrome" trigger. Although there's often overlap between the terms, when people's reactions to toxins are limited to a specific building, the designation "sick building syndrome" is often used. Once the reactions no longer clear when the people leave the building in question, they can be said to have chemical sensitivity. Taylor shares a building-related story of developing chemical illness as a child.

> I first realized I had MCS when I was ten and in the sixth grade. We moved to a brand-new school, and I got so sick every day that I would throw up several times before first hour was over. Of course, doctors didn't want to believe that something was making me sick and kept telling me that I just didn't want to go to school. I had a battery of allergy tests done, which made me ill, but all came back negative, and the allergist said that it was psychosomatic.

> After doing a lot of research on our own, my parents determined that I had MCS. They took me out of the school and started homeschooling me. I started feeling better after being out of the building for a while and loved homeschooling. I was relatively healthy because I stayed away from toxins as much as possible.

Common chemicals and possible exposure symptoms. The list of possible chemical exposures and resultant health effects is enormous. The Environmental Protection Agency (EPA) lists the following effects of some common chemicals.[41] The list only scratches the surface of possible exposures and symptoms.

- Benzene occurs in glues, paints, furniture wax, vehicle exhaust, cigarette smoke, and many other sources. Studies link it to bronchitis, blood cell changes, dizziness, vomiting, eye and skin irritation, asthma, leukemia, and Hodgkin's lymphoma.

- Formaldehyde is a very common substance found in pressed wood products, carpet, foam insulation, cosmetics, cleaning products, some finger paints and nail hardeners, and many other places. Among its health effects are asthma, inflammation and toxicity of the intestinal tract, cancer of the respiratory tract, and irritation of the respiratory tract, skin, and eyes.

- TCE (trichloroethylene) occurs in glues, varnish and paint removers, and vinyl flooring. It can cause arthritis; high blood pressure; anemia; headaches; dizziness; confusion; liver, kidney, immunological, endocrine and respiratory problems; and several cancers.

- Exposure to Benzo(a)pyrene (BaP) occurs from wood stoves, tar and asphalt fumes, and car exhaust, among other places. Research links it to altered DNA replication, cancer, and immune system effects.

- Vinyl chloride, a component of vinyl and plastics, may cause dizziness, drowsiness, headaches, giddiness, and some cancers.

- Various forms of mercury can be found in fluorescent bulbs, thermometers, dental amalgam fillings, vaccine preservatives, fish, older paint, some health remedies, creams, batteries, disinfectants, and antiseptics. The long list of health effects includes behavioral changes, tremors, reduced muscle coordination, leg cramps, peeling skin, itching, fever, sweating, salivating, rashes, sleeplessness, weakness, renal and pulmonary toxicity, hypertension, diarrhea, nausea, ulcers, increased blood pressure, decreased heart rate variability, twitching, tics, impaired gait, miscarriage, stillbirths and birth defects, effects on attention, fine motor function, language, visual-spatial abilities, and verbal memory.

- Arsenic may be found in water, soil, and some wood preservatives. It can cause nausea, diarrhea, abdominal pain, skin effects, and many cancers.

- Nitrates and nitrites are common components of gasoline, shoe polish, spray paints, fertilizers, rat poison, and food preservatives.

They can cause abdominal pain, muscle weakness, fainting, spleen hemorrhaging, increased risk of childhood diabetes, recurrent diarrhea, and recurrent respiratory tract infections. Fetal exposure is associated with increased risk of sudden infant death syndrome (SIDS) and cardiac and nervous system defects.

Pesticides (the term includes herbicides) are specifically designed to kill, which is, of course, what the "cide" suffix means, and therefore are potentially very dangerous. In fact, the poison used to kill prisoners in the gas chambers of Auschwitz was a pesticide.[42] Children who live in homes where pesticides are used are twice as likely to develop brain cancer.[43]

Further effects of some common pesticides sold today include the following:

- 2, 4-D occurs in over 1,500 pesticide products, is often used on residential lawns, and is frequently found in the dust of homes and other buildings. Studies link it to blood, liver, and kidney toxicity, coughing, a burning sensation in the lungs, loss of muscular coordination, nausea, vomiting, and dizziness.

- Atrazine, an herbicide often used on golf courses, roadway grasses, and residential lawns, frequently occurs in drinking water. It is an endocrine disruptor with effects on hormones, the central nervous system, and the immune system. Atrazine exposure increases the risk of non-Hodgkin's lymphoma and preterm delivery and decreased birth weight of newborns.

- DDVP (Dichlorvos) can be found in flea collars, pest strips, pesticide sprays, and foggers. It affects the brain, plasma, and red blood cells and can cause nausea, anxiousness, restlessness, teary eyes, heavy sweating, and many cancers.

- Pyrethroids are generally used in lice shampoos, pet flea shampoos, household foggers, and municipal mosquito abatement products. Exposure can cause dizziness, twitching, nervous disorders, skin and respiratory irritation, and immunotoxic effects.

Studies have found many other chemical/body reactions not commonly associated. *The Washington Post* reported that a number of researchers believe certain chemicals can trigger fat-cell activity and contribute to obesity.[44] In the same vein, Ashford and Miller note that insatiable hunger or food cravings may be a withdrawal symptom from certain chemical exposures. They also note that increased blood pressure, heart rate, and arrhythmias are attributed to the wearing of synthetic clothing versus cotton, that panic disorder has been associated with organic solvent exposure and that avoidance of smoking improved psychosis in some schizophrenic patients, while rechallenge exacerbated it.[45] A surprising study found that children who live in homes with vinyl floors are twice as likely to have autism, a connection that one of the study authors said "turned up virtually by accident."[46] Undoubtedly, a vast number of similar connections await discovery.

Take Care Tips

- Begin to make changes in the products you use. If you feel overwhelmed, remind yourself that it isn't necessary to change everything at once. Just take a step, then take another.

- Replace toxic items such as cleaning, personal care, yard and garden, and pest control products with nontoxic alternatives. Some items don't need to be replaced, but simply removed. Synthetically fragranced "air fresheners," for example, fall into this category. There is nothing fresher than clean, pure air.

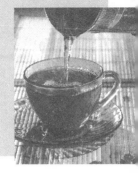

DOESN'T THE GOVERNMENT PROTECT US?

It's common and reassuring to think the government is safeguarding our health and won't allow the sale of truly harmful products. The truth, however, is that we're part of an ongoing experiment in which chemical products are making their way to our store shelves without ever being tested for human health effects. Take, for example, the ubiquitous formulations generally labeled simply "fragrance." Many people believe the FDA (Food and Drug Administration) regulates cosmetics and other personal care products. However, cosmetics are neither foods nor drugs and simply aren't tested the way a drug would be. An MSNBC article notes that, "essentially, protection lies in the hands of the fragrance industry."[47]

Just what is "fragrance" anyway? In the past, manufacturers made perfumes from natural ingredients. That's certainly no longer the case. An article in *Environmental Health Perspectives*, a journal published by the National Institute of Environmental Health Sciences, notes that it's estimated that more than three thousand chemicals are used in the manufacture of fragrances and that a single fragrance may contain as many as several hundred chemicals.[48] What kinds of chemicals? The National Academy of Sciences states that 95 percent come from petroleum. These include known toxins capable of causing cancer, birth defects, central nervous system disorders, and allergic reactions.[49]

The chemical problem goes far beyond fragrances, of course. Multiply the "fragrance" situation many times over to include building products, cleaning supplies, yard and garden chemicals, and much more, and the extent of the problem becomes more apparent. Currently there are about 80,000 chemicals registered for use in the USA, with more than 2,000 new chemicals introduced each year.[50] Of those 80,000 chemicals, the Environmental Protection Agency (EPA) has required testing of two hundred[51] and regulates five.[52]

Alex notes:

> I'm just like everyone else, I guess, and used to think that if it was sold on the shelf that it was safe. It's been completely shocking to me to discover how completely unregulated all this stuff is. It's like the Wild West.

An *LA Times* article by Al Meyerhoff pointed out that the lack of testing leads to "what is charitably called the 'data gap'—a paucity of information about the toxicity of these products and the effects of our exposure to them." The article also noted that "these 'gaps' are not a secret. They were supposed to be filled more than thirty years ago when Congress passed a woefully inadequate law called the Toxic Substances Control Act."[53]

After decades of inaction, there's been a bit of forward progress in the regulatory realm. The awkwardly-named Frank R. Lautenberg Chemical Safety for the 21st Century Act was signed into law in June of 2016. It gives the Environmental Protection Agency some new ability to address the issue of toxic products. Although it's a step in the right direction, one organization involved with the issue concluded that "The pace of change will be slow. . . . There are some unnecessary activities required that will divert resources and there are some loopholes in the law."[54] In other words, we can be grateful for forward motion but will have to continue to be diligent and smart about what we buy and use.

Limitations of testing and labeling. The fact that very few products are tested for toxicity is only part of the problem. Even the products tested for safety are generally not tested in combination with other products (in other words, not tested in the lab the way people will use them in real life). One popular ulcer medication, for example, can make a person a hundred to a thousand times more sensitive to the poisoning effects of organophosphates, compounds commonly found in insecticides, herbicides, and fertilizers.[55]

Linda Birnbaum notes that some chemicals may act in an additive fashion. She points out that a chemical often found in plastics mimics estrogen in the body and could be acting synergistically with other pseudoestrogens to produce heart disease, diabetes, or liver failure. Animal studies demonstrate such effects. Birnbaum states, "When we look at one compound at a time, we may miss the boat."[56]

In one study, biologists tested four herbicides, two fungicides, and three insecticides commonly used in American cornfields. On their own, the chemicals had little effect on developing tadpoles when the exposure level was low. But when they were exposed to all nine chemicals at the same low level in the laboratory—the lowest level actually found in the field—the tadpoles developed infection, took longer to mature, and a third of them died.[57]

Animal studies can be instructive, but they're an imperfect means of determining human danger. Donohoe notes that "we have made the world safer for rats and other test species than we have for humans." He adds:

> Every day in my practice I see people who, had they been rats, would not be sick. They had the dreadful misfortune to be humans in a rat's world. They expose themselves to chemicals at doses rats would be fine with and develop asthma, brain damage, immune disorders, cancers, infertility, damage to the chromosomes, and more. Many, tragically, die.[58]

Another testing problem is the fact that risk assessment often focuses on a narrow range of effects. Pesticide testing is an example. Lawson notes that most pesticides are nerve poisons, but the EPA doesn't test them for effects on the nervous and immune systems.[59]

Labeling is another area that lacks regulation. A single benign-sounding word or two can hide many toxins. Toxins can also be present in items due to the breakdown of other ingredients. For example, the Campaign for Safe Cosmetics tested a number of children's bath products for two cancer-causing chemicals and found that 67 percent contained one of them, 82 percent contained the other, and 61 percent contained both, although no labels listed either substance. The chemicals are considered "contaminants" rather than "ingredients" and are exempt from labeling laws.[60]

Another favorite labeling trick is to "greenwash" a product by including words like "natural" or "green" in an item's title or on its label. These terms are used indiscriminately, have very little meaning, and can be quite misleading. The term "green" is especially problematic. A green product is purported to be better for the environment than standard fare, but better for the environment doesn't necessarily mean better for human health. Recycling a toxic product, for example, doesn't make it less toxic. Although labels don't tell the whole story of a product's chemical dangers, there are sometimes clues such as the warning to keep a product out of the reach of children or the instruction to read safety directions before using.

Who's in charge? There are many government agencies. Surely, one can fill the gaps left by another, right? That wasn't the experience of Lorraine

Smith. Smith was a teacher, and when workers put a new roof on her school building, she became very ill.

In an attempt to protect the students in the building and learn what chemicals were used, Smith first called the roofing company and could get no answers. She then called the Occupational Safety and Health Agency (OSHA). They told her they only had jurisdiction over the private sector and had no say in the school system. She was told to call her state Department of Education, but when she did, she was amazed to learn they had no regulations or safety codes for air quality in the schools. Finally, she called the Division of Occupational Hygiene and learned they did not intend to check the situation. She writes, "I could not find a single agency to help. I kept thinking of the children breathing those fumes. . . ."[61]

Regulations regarding testing, labeling, and toxin emissions are important. In some cases, new laws are needed and in others, existing laws need to be enforced. It's also vitally important that we each take responsibility for what we buy and use. Ultimately, God calls each of us to be stewards of our own health and to care for those around us affected by the product choices we make.

Take Care Tips

- Don't assume that something is safe because it's for sale. Take responsibility for understanding the toxicity of the products you use.

- Remember that "green" is an imprecise and evolving term that may mean a product is better for the environment in some way, but it doesn't necessarily mean it's better for human health. Look for products designed with human safety in mind.

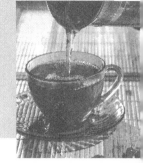

$\mathcal{S}$earch

Cry out for insight and ask for understanding.
Search for them as you would for silver;
seek them like hidden treasures.
—Proverbs 2:3–4

When people realize they're ill and not recovering, they move into the second stage on the journey of chemical illness—the *Search* phase. Sufferers are searching for diagnoses and for more relief than they're getting from the over-the-counter treatments they've been using. Their symptoms have become too insistent to ignore and are interfering too much with their daily lives. The types of doctors seen in this phase and the diagnoses received vary as much as sufferers' symptoms do. Sometimes people enter this phase with a clue that chemical exposures are part of their problem, but often they have no idea.

DIAGNOSIS PROGNOSIS

One of the first problems with diagnosis is that people with symptoms caused by chemical exposures will often pass standard lab tests. To be useful, tests need the correct focus. If someone has a broken leg, for example, an x-ray of the arm won't reveal the problem. Stories like the following are typical:

I was very ill and felt like I was dying. I had been working in a newly remodeled building that was poorly ventilated. My doctor ran tests on me including an MRI. All he found was that my liver enzymes were up.

———————•••◦•◦•◦———————

As the severity of my symptoms increased, I began regular visits to doctors' offices, emergency rooms, and urgent care facilities. But they were looking for disease, and I was experiencing poisoning. They were never going to understand what was making me sick.[62]

When one test isn't helpful, it's logical to move onto another and then another. Unfortunately, extensive testing tends to be expensive testing. Parker relates a common scenario.

I had to spend so much time, energy, and money proving what I didn't have before the doctor would really believe that it was MCS. I spent $17,000 out-of-pocket. The tests with dye in them made the MCS worse. It was difficult doing all that testing.

"No problem found" lab tests can lead to self-doubt, prolonged suffering, and a long parade of doctors and exams. Although helpful lab tests may be rare at this stage, diagnoses are not. Kendall remembers the journey.

I was told: "It must be Parkinson's since you swung your leg and bobbed your head." Another doctor said my diabetes was out of control. I wasn't diabetic.

Any illness can be misdiagnosed. A study published in the *Journal of the American Medical Association* reported that autopsy studies find that doctors are wrong 10 to 15 percent of the time.[63] The rate of misdiagnoses is undoubtedly higher, though, when related to subjects not generally covered thoroughly in medical training. The Association of American Medical

Colleges reports that one quarter of medical schools don't require their students to learn any environmental medicine, and of those who do, students receive only seven hours of training.[64]

Other factors may contribute to misdiagnosis as well. I once read a somewhat tongue-in-cheek theory that the doctors who make it through medical school with their health intact after exposure to chemicals in their training are those with extra-strong detoxification systems and are the least likely to be aware of chemical effects or sympathetic to patients who experience them. Chapter 8 discusses a more serious reason for ignorance and misinformation about toxic illness in the medical field.

When the *Search* phase begins, patients generally trust their doctors and believe in the diagnoses they receive. If doctors prescribe medications, patients take them. Sufferers want to get well and have no reason to doubt they will.

The problem with medications for the chemically ill is that most are synthetic creations that rely on the same detoxification pathways that are already damaged. Although some with toxic illness have found helpful drugs, people reactive to chemicals are often medication-intolerant. If there are possible side effects, chemical illness sufferers are likely to experience them in large degree. People in the *Search* phase thus find themselves not only failing to improve, but often getting significantly worse. A study that asked chemically reactive people about treatments they had tried, and whether they were helpful, found that prescription drugs had the lowest efficacy ratings, with many rated more likely to harm than help.[65]

Take Care Tip

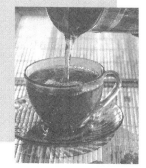

- If you or people you know are suffering from unexplained health symptoms, don't dismiss or minimize the problem if doctors can't immediately pinpoint the cause or provide a quick solution. Be open to the idea that chemical toxicity may be playing a role.

Stress and Distress

The types of diagnoses received in the *Search* phase vary widely, but often the first one given is "stress." People with chemical illness have found some solace in the knowledge that many diseases have been blamed on stress, including ulcers, asthma, Crohn's disease, and cancer.[66]

> The eye specialist kept saying my problem was "stress." For years he said that. Stress is a good diagnosis for what you don't have an answer for.

> As soon as a doctor asks, "Have you been under a lot of pressure lately?" my heart just sinks. I've learned from experience that whether I say "yes" or "no" doesn't matter. Either way I'll be told my problems are due to stress and that's as far as the diagnosis process will go.

It's absolutely true that stress of various kinds can affect the immune system and other body processes and predispose people to various illnesses. Emotional stress can have definite physical ramifications. It's just that "stress" isn't the full story, even when it's part of it. Unfortunately, once the body is damaged, removing the stress doesn't automatically fix the problems any more than a good night's sleep will repair the injuries of someone who had a car wreck from falling asleep at the wheel or removing the bullet will fix the internal injuries of someone who has been shot.

Intended or not, a stress diagnosis seems to carry a connotation of blame. No matter what doctors actually mean when they blame stress for an illness, what patients tend to hear is, "You got yourself into this by not managing your life well, and you should be able to get yourself out of it too." A diagnosis of stress can be stressful.

Searching for causes in all the wrong places. Another thing chemically ill patients often hear is that their symptoms are psychosomatic in nature, or they have some version of hypochondria, paranoia, or another mental illness.

The journal *COJ Nursing and Healthcare* reports on a family of four who all became ill after moving to a new home in the country.

> Years of hospitalisations, scans, pathology tests, and exploratory surgery having produced only negative results, the mother, the worst affected, was eventually labelled psychosomatic. Not for thirteen years, until admitted to an ECU—a hospital ward stripped of all potential reactive agents—was her condition correctly diagnosed. Blinded placebo-controlled challenge testing revealed that every symptom so long attributed to stress was in fact a manifestation of environmental sensitivity.[67]

Lisa relates some of the advice and diagnoses she received in the *Search* phase.

> "There is nothing wrong with you. Go and beg for your job back!"

> "Get some counseling for the grief."

> "Quit talking about it, and you'll get better."

> "Ignore it, and suck it up."

> "You just want attention, and you want to make people take care of you." (My family got a good laugh from that one—since I am "Miss Independence.")

> "Obsessive compulsive to perfume."

> "Unresolved issues from childhood."

Unfortunately, such treatment seems the norm rather than the exception. Others share their experiences of searching for help from the medical profession.

I was one of those people that had no clue until it was too late. I just accepted them saying I was a hypochondriac.

I worked as a mental health counselor for fifteen years. I started having problems with MCS after the agency I worked for bought an old store and made a counseling center out of it. The only windows were in the front of the building and my office was in the middle. A few months after I moved in, I started having symptoms I couldn't explain such as racing heart, panic attacks, brain fog, mini seizures, joint and muscle pain, depression, and headaches. I went to my doctor who told me he couldn't find anything wrong with me. The psychiatrist I worked with said I was just like all the postmenopausal women he knew and gave me antidepressants and benzos. I took them so I could continue working, but the side effects were so great I had to quit them. I couldn't keep up with my job, and my mind and energy slowed down. I had to quit the job I loved.

The general population views certain hospitals and clinics as better than others at diagnosing and treating difficult medical cases. It's not unusual for desperate people to travel long distances in search of answers there. Allie's story involves a trip to a well-known hospital.

I went to my GP for the stomach problems, hands going numb, etc. I was also having terrible headaches and was concerned I might have a brain tumor or something terrible like that. I didn't mention MCS but just tried to tell her my symptoms, and she refused to listen. All she wanted to focus on was the weight I had lost, which wasn't that much at first. I have always been a small person and was not unhealthily thin when I started going to her. My doctor told me that I was anorexic despite my insistence that I did eat, did not make myself throw up, and did not want to lose weight. She said that she could give me an antidepressant to stimulate my appetite. I went to doctor after doctor during that spring, trying to find someone to find what was wrong. I suspected MCS, but I was even hesitant to believe it because everyone wanted "proof."

Finally, my parents decided to listen to everyone and take me to a well-known clinic generally regarded as "the best." It was the most traumatic, most awful experience I have ever had. I still have nightmares about it. They lied and said that they didn't have a diagnosis but would admit me for extensive tests when, in reality, they admitted me for anorexia. The only doctor who came to see me was a psychiatrist, not all of the specialists that they had promised. The place was filthy and noisy and the doctors and nurses were rude to me and treated me like a prisoner. I felt so sick that I could hardly hold my head up and the brain fog was the worst I had ever experienced. Somehow, I managed to have the strength to understand what was going on and what their plans were (to institutionalize me) though my parents had not yet figured it out.

The first night in the hospital, I suffered the worst/most terrifying reaction ever. My tongue swelled so huge that it took up my entire mouth, and I was gasping for breath. I literally believe that I almost died. I remember feeling blackness sweeping over me as I struggled to get air. My parents had not left for the night yet and called the doctor, who was a clueless intern. She said I was having a panic attack. My mom figured things out by then and realized that it was the MCS. When she told the doctor that, she had never even heard of it.

Dad kept telling me that I had to give it one more day. I remember crying and begging him to take me home, insisting that I was going to die if I stayed there. After more lying on the part of the doctors, I somehow scraped together my mental faculties enough to refuse tests that I had already had, which had made me extremely sick. Dad finally realized what they had admitted me for and that they weren't going to help. We packed up and got out of there. The doctors were very reluctant to let me leave, and there were a few terrifying minutes when I thought they were going to keep me there against my will.

I've read stories from other toxic illness sufferers about doctors indeed keeping them against their will and confining them to psychiatric wards where their symptoms predictably continued to worsen.

Dr. Mark Donohoe, who works with the chemically ill, speaks directly to the issue of "crazy people, crazy doctors." He writes:

> Where causes are not easily found, we invent causes. The brief is simple—invented causes need to be unprovable and disprovable. They need to give the impression of science. They need to make the majority of us comfortable that the causes do not apply to us. We need, in short, a type of rubbish bin for medicine, where we dump the conditions and people who we either do not understand, or who make us uncomfortable. Psychology and psychiatry will do for now.[68]

Dr. Pamela Gibson reported that over half of the chemically reactive people she surveyed received mental illness labels including "olfactory delusions" (related to being able to smell things others could not) or even schizophrenia based on those "delusions."[69]

It isn't impossible, of course, for those with toxic illness to have coexisting psychological disorders, or for chemical exposures to cause psychological symptoms. Alison Johnson points out that mercury in the felt they used probably made the "Mad Hatters" of the nineteenth century insane.[70] It's also theoretically possible that certain isolated cases of environmental illness are indeed psychological.

Those truths, however, don't negate the fact that chemical illness is a very real physical condition. When a woman experiences pseudocyesis, she believes she's pregnant, though she's not, and sometimes she even manifests some physical signs. Pseudocyesis exists, but that doesn't mean that pregnancy isn't a real, physical condition, and it certainly doesn't mean that the great majority of women who believe they're pregnant are mentally ill. Too often, in the case of chemical injury, a psychiatric diagnosis seems to be the default "go-to" explanation that stops all further investigation.

Sometimes clinicians diagnose people with chemical illness with agoraphobia, having a fear of crowds or public places. Johnson notes that diagnosis is "tantamount to saying to a paraplegic in a wheelchair, 'Too bad you don't like to walk.'"[71] Johnson also points out that critics often claim that "secondary gain" is a strong component of the condition. The theory is that sufferers act as they do because they want others to care for them. She states that

> One does not have to read too many of the stories [of chemically reactive people] before it is apparent that this suggestion is at best made in ignorance, and at worst represents an exceedingly cruel attitude toward people whose illness has in all too many cases cost them their job, their home, their friends, or their spouse.[72]

She notes that patients who react to medications may be accused of overtly resisting treatment, making the secondary gain diagnosis more likely.

The secondary gain hypothesis is easy to apply. Timothy, profiled in *Casualties of Progress*, was a healthy four-year-old when his parents installed new carpet in their home. First he developed a cough, then breathing difficulties, then loss of cognitive function, then severe vomiting. His mother writes:

> Within a few days Timothy had become so sick that I had to carry him upstairs and to the bathroom. He didn't have the strength to walk, and his arms hurt, and his joints hurt. He would just curl up in a fetal position and lie on the couch. When I told this to Timothy's doctor, he told me that Timothy was playing mind games with me and that he wasn't sick. He said that Timothy just didn't want to walk to the bathroom. He told me he thought Timothy was lazy

and that he should get up and get moving. And this is a four-year-old we're talking about.[73]

It's not only doctors who diagnose. It isn't only doctors who mistake toxic illness for a psychological disorder. Pastor and radio host Jim Andrews, in his book *Polishing God's Monuments*, speaks of his daughter Juli's struggle with Chronic Fatigue Syndrome and MCS. He tells of a "well-intentioned, but woefully uninformed and egregiously misguided lady" who formed a support group for Andrews and his wife and invited them to the first meeting. At the meeting, she presented them with a book on panic attacks and announced that she'd arranged an appointment for Juli with a psychiatrist. Andrews notes that "this lady had never seen Juli, never asked us about Juli, had almost no specific knowledge of her symptoms, yet made up her own mind about the nature of her condition."[74]

An ironic story in Johnson's book is of David, a practicing psychologist with a PhD. When chemical illness forced him to quit work, family members evidently decided they'd learned enough psychology from the doctor to diagnose him. They decided he was having a midlife crisis, called him a malingerer, and concluded the condition was all in his head.[75] Christa Upton in her book *MCS: Banished from the Human Race,* sums up how it feels.

> In the worst time of your life, often when you cannot take care of your family and/or work to support your family, having people blame your Multiple Chemical Sensitivity and resulting devastating problems on you is something that rips at your very being.[76]

The truth is that most people just don't think of looking to chemicals in the everyday environment as a cause for health-related problems. Even when doctors or others haven't given wrong diagnoses, people are capable of coming up with all sorts of theories on their own. Donna shares her experience with perfume-related brain effects.

> I was talking with my new step-mother-in-law, and I could not remember basic words like the word car. I could think of what I was trying to say, but I could not find any words

to say it. The more I was around this woman, the worse it got. [Eventually] when I was near her, I could no longer even think of anything at all to say; it was like someone had taken an eraser to my brain. My husband and I joked that it was the ghost of Millie, my deceased mother-in-law. Without joking, I wondered if I felt so ambivalent about having a new mother-in-law that it prevented me from being able to speak. The temptation to resort to simple psychological explanations for physiological problems induced by chemical injury is great indeed. It turns out that when my step-mother-in-law does not wear her favorite brand of designer perfume, I have plenty of things to say. Clearly not ambivalent feelings, but chemicals.[77]

Michael, another "casualty of progress" profiled in Johnson's book, relates his experience with toxic illness and church attendance. In his case, physical symptoms caused by chemicals led him to a spiritual conclusion. He states:

Judy and I have always gone to church. In fact, on our first date we went to church before we went to dinner. . . . When I started getting sick, before I realized what was going on, I noticed that when I went to church I would be really ill before the service was over, if I could even make it through the service. Sometimes I literally had to stumble out of church because I felt so ill. I thought I had done something bad . . . and God was throwing me out of church. I really was concerned about what was going on.[78]

Dealing with the ongoing symptoms. Especially for those in the *Search* phase who don't have a clue about the chemical/symptom connection, a diagnosis of "crazy or stressed" often prompts very mixed emotions. Sufferers feel relieved that they haven't been diagnosed with anything life threatening, but they're often embarrassed that they can't seem to manage their lives well enough to stay healthy and ashamed to tell others what the medical professionals have told them. They try to downplay their struggles in a desire to remain "normal" or to not appear weak. They push through life with forced smiles and feel like they're drowning.

The *Search* phase can be extremely difficult. Sufferers are having severe symptoms, but the doctors' suggestions aren't helping at all, and in many instances are making things worse. Medical bills are piling up, and everyone is expecting daily activities to continue at full speed. The fact that many chemical and food reactions can be emotional in nature (causing depression, rage, etc.) and that sufferers don't yet know to avoid those triggers, makes this an especially tense and emotional stage.

The lack of understanding can cause much relationship discord. Flora Preston, in her book *Convenient, "Safe" and Deadly*, writes that she knew she was ill, but that her doctors couldn't diagnose her, which led to friction between her and her roommates. She notes:

> Cleaning the bathroom exhausted me, but I had lots of energy to play soccer. What I did not know was that I was reacting to the cleansers I was using to clean the bathroom. I might clean the bathtub and then need to rest for a half-hour before I had the energy and muscle strength to clean the rest of the bathroom. The fact I had lots of energy to play soccer after I had some more rest really added to the confusion. . . . Since I did not know I was reacting to the cleansers, I could not share that with my roommates. All I could say was that I did not understand, either.[79]

Sufferers typically feel very misunderstood and alone in the *Search* phase and are desperate for help. Some typical scenarios:

> It was the most horrible time in my life. I kept getting sicker and sicker and losing more weight. People were cruel and constantly on my back that I just needed to eat more. Everyone who I thought would support me didn't. Every doctor's visit made me sicker. I eventually determined that

one of the biggest triggers for my MCS is doctors' and dentists' sterile equipment and office buildings.

When I look back at the time when I was already sick, but didn't know why, I can still remember how truly, truly, awful it was. Just to get through the day was like running a marathon or fighting a war. I had young children, and I gave them every ounce of energy I could possibly find inside me, which left me with absolutely nothing in reserve. The pain level was incredible and it never, ever, let up. The worst part was being so incredibly sick, but getting no support from anyone. No one seemed to have the time or inclination to even listen to me, much less believe the extent of the problem. I felt like everyone just wanted me to keep my mouth shut and do what they needed me to do, and I've never felt so undervalued, alone, and completely desperate in my life. Somehow, by the grace of God, I managed to get through that time with my marriage, family, and sanity intact, but I would never, ever, ever want to go through that again.

It's not uncommon for people describing their time in the *Search* phase to say they thought they were going to die. Others describe feeling like they're about to go over a cliff or shatter into pieces. "Fragile" is the way I remember feeling (a designation that one doctor seemed to somehow take as a personal affront). The phase can vary greatly in duration. Some people are fortunate to receive a diagnosis quickly, but others search for an answer for years, while symptoms continue to worsen, as the following experiences illustrate:

I have had MCS for thirty-three years and just found out three years ago.

I didn't know that I had MCS. I describe it like driving down the road and the "dead end" sign is missing. I went plowing off the edge, and my life as I knew it was over. Many people can lead good, active lives by avoiding extra exposure. I can't now, and I don't want people to end up like me.

Take Care Tips

- Avoid jumping to the conclusion that an unexplained illness is psychological.

- Don't let diagnoses such as stress, depression, or hypochondria shut the door on considering other options. If chemicals play a role in the symptom picture, the sooner people discover and address the issue, the better the chances are for a full recovery.

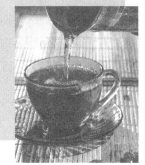

THE MOMENT OF DISCOVERY

Chemically ill people become aware of the connection between chemicals and their symptoms in a variety of ways. A survey found that when asked who initially identified their condition, the largest percentage of participants (34%) reported identifying the problem themselves. Over a quarter of the participants (26%) received diagnoses from health providers, while 6 percent said a friend or family member identified the problem, 4 percent were helped by the media, and 29 percent said that it was some combination of the above.[80]

Those helped by the media evidently don't need hand holding. My favorite diagnosis story is of a woman who watched a television news report that portrayed MCS in a negative light, but she recognized the symptoms and excitedly told her husband she knew what was wrong with them now.[81] Sometimes a small bit of information can allow all the puzzle pieces to fall into place.

It's not always that easy to make the connection. Angela Cummings writes about her journey. She states that during eight years of searching, five of her doctors and six of her son's doctors were unable to diagnose their problems. Three doctors told her they were out of ideas and told her to figure it out. She writes:

> I was left to my own devices to do just that—figure it out. After [studying] four inches of medical records and analyzing its contents, I could see the pattern of infection rise and fall when we were living outside of our house for a period of time. The cause became clear. Our new home was causing life-changing medical issues.[82]

At times, doctors point patients in the right direction without actually giving a firm diagnosis. My own journey of discovery began when a doctor suggested a restricted diet, which improved my health greatly but didn't relieve all my symptoms. One day he offhandedly said, "Well, maybe you should also avoid detergent." Detergent? I was living in Peru then and half-wondered if maybe I had misunderstood him because of language issues. The suggestion seemed nonsensical, but it began the research and experimentation that eventually allowed me to understand what caused my symptoms (a lot more than detergent, unfortunately) and how to reduce them.

Others share their stories.

> My doctor has never officially said to me, "You have MCS." Because the medical profession at large generally doesn't recognize that diagnosis, many doctors don't come right out and say it. Each doctor wants to call our diagnosis something different.

I discovered my sensitivity to chemicals after the apartments had all been sprayed heavily with pesticides. When I couldn't touch my couch, or anything that had previously touched my couch for that matter, without breaking out into a rash, I found a book at the library called Toxic House or something like that, and it all made sense to me and paralleled what I was experiencing.

I found out I had MCS two and a half years ago. I found out from the internet. I don't remember the search word I entered, but it pulled up "Chemical Sensitivity." It was about 10:30 p.m., and I just sat there and cried with joy. It had a name. I wanted to call my daughter but her family was in bed. I had been told that it was in my head for so many years that I was stunned to find all my illness pointed to one diagnosis—MCS.

When people make the connection, the *Search* phase ends and the *Sift* phase begins.

Take Care Tips

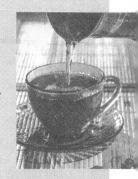

- If you suspect you may have chemical illness, continue to educate yourself about the issue, and immediately begin reducing the level of toxins in your environment. If you suspect toxic illness in others, provide them with information without being pushy or dogmatic.

- Help searchers find doctors who are tuned into chemical issues. See the resource section at the end of this book for help.

CHAPTER THREE

Sift

A prudent person foresees danger and takes precautions.
—Proverbs 22:3

The *Sift* phase begins when people realize, to their great relief, that they can control their symptoms to a large degree by avoiding triggering chemicals. They begin to sift through the products that surround them to determine what to keep and what to discard. They're thrilled to find some abatement of symptoms and relieved to discover some control over their health. Because chemicals in the environment are sickening all people to some degree, it's prudent for everyone to engage in the sifting process and transition to a less toxic life.

Although avoiding toxins is important for everyone, some people may have extra motivation to address the issue. The knowledge that their bodies are temples of the Holy Spirit should inspire Christians to take the topic seriously.[83] Parents of young children should also be especially careful because little bodies detoxify smaller amounts of toxins than larger bodies do. Those suffering more severe symptoms tend to want to make changes more than those who feel generally healthy, but I hope more knowledge about the consequences of exceeding a body's detoxification capacity will motivate those in that category.

In general, chemically reactive people are confident in the *Sift* phase that if they isolate themselves from chemical exposures for a while their bodies will heal. For many in the early stages of toxic illness, small changes do indeed bring much improvement. The challenge of this phase is that avoiding offending chemicals is much easier in theory than it is in practice. A broad overview of some of the challenges and general principles follows.

FORGOING FRAGRANCE

A relatively easy way to begin the sifting process is to focus on personal care products, especially those that affect not only the users but those around them. Synthetic fragrances are some of the most obvious problematic chemicals in this category. If good health and caring for others are goals, people should refrain from using modern perfumes, colognes, or other lab-created concoctions designed simply to provide an artificial fragrance. They should replace synthetically-scented items such as shampoo, conditioner, lotion, makeup, shaving cream, and soap with fragrance-free alternatives.

Fortunately, fragrance-free products are much easier to find in mainstream stores than they once were, and the more people buy them, the more available they'll become. Every purchase of a less-toxic product not only benefits the purchasers and those around them, but also sends a message to the manufacturers about what consumers prefer to find on the shelves. Of course, there can be many other problematic ingredients in personal care products besides synthetic fragrances, but becoming fragrance-free is an easy way to lower the toxic load. (See the resource list for product database tools and sources for healthier choices.)

Sometimes people who don't feel the need to make changes for their own health become aware of the sensitivities of others around them, and they kindly attempt to be fragrance-free on those occasions when they know they'll be seeing the sufferer. Unfortunately, most people have no idea how truly pervasive synthetic fragrances are. The average person applies twelve fragranced products a day.[84] To the user, the scent may seem minimal, due to olfactory fatigue (the inability to distinguish an odor after prolonged exposure to it), but to the chemically ill it can be overpowering and dangerous.

Laundry products. When people begin making changes, they can easily overlook many sources of synthetic fragrance. Laundry products, for example, can cause significant problems.

Toxic illness sufferers share some laundry-related experiences.

At church-related small group meetings, the ladies would say, "I'm not wearing perfume," but I could tell they washed and dried their clothes in fragranced products. People just are not aware how permeated our society is with scented stuff.

My library group agreed to not wear perfume, but I ended up sitting next to someone who was using the detergent that's worst for me. My daughter laughed when I told her the gal next to me uses that brand. She asked how I could possibly know. I said, "Because of the way it burns my eyes, nose, and throat. Go ahead, ask her." Sure enough, I was right. Nasty stuff.

Having to explain everything is so much work. I found with home Bible study that I was being exposed to fabric softeners—some from use in the home and some from the people coming to the group. I tried but had to give it up.

People with chemical illness find themselves attending social events less and less often. Even hosting visitors in their own safe homes can be difficult. People unknowingly bring chemicals into the home that linger, often contaminating previously safe items and making the home less safe.

It's common for visitors to believe that washing their clothes in a fragrance-free detergent before coming to visit will take care of the problem. Unfortunately, synthetic fragrances are *extremely* difficult to remove, and if an item has had a fragranced detergent or fabric softener used on it, it may take months of repeated washings in a safe product before the item can even approach chemical safety. Often the item can never be redeemed.

A chemical illness sufferer once called a major dryer sheet manufacturer to ask how to remove the residue. The spokesperson told her that the company designed the product to bond with fabric permanently and to never release. Never is a long time. It's similar to how dyed cloth is unlikely to return to its former color. Even when people stop using dryer sheets and buy new clothing, the residual chemicals from the sheets have often coated the dryer and to some extent will contaminate whatever else is inside.

It's emotionally difficult on both sides when people try hard to make accommodations for the chemically sensitive, but the efforts fall short, as the following example shows.

> One of my favorite people came over to visit last week. She changed her detergent a few months ago to try to make herself safe for me, but there was enough residual fragrance in her clothes that I became immediately ill. I've been in bed since her visit and, as much as I love her, I don't think I want her to come back.

Typical laundry products can be problematic for everyone in their vicinity, but are of special concern for those wearing the affected clothes. The chemicals coat the items and are continually absorbed into the body when the clothing is worn. Human skin is porous, which is why topical medications work.

Many household products are heavily fragranced because manufacturers add the fragrance to cover the odor of other toxic chemicals. Dryer sheets are a prime example. Most brands contain many strong chemicals known to be carcinogenic and cause central nervous system disorders. One of the chemicals used is actually on the EPA's hazardous waste list.[85] One author notes, "The chemicals in fabric softeners are pungent and strong smelling—so strong that they require the use of these heavy fragrances (think fifty times as much fragrance) just to cover up the smells. Furthermore, synthetic fabrics, which are the reason fabric softeners were created in the first place, do not smell good either when heated in a dryer or heated by our bodies . . . hence the need for even more hefty fragrances."[86]

Although I've never seen an official poll on the issue, I've been in several forums where the chemically ill have been asked what single product they would ban if they could, and dryer sheets were a very common answer. They're unnecessary, and those who wish to take the best possible care of the body of Christ, both in an individual and corporate sense, should avoid them.

Take Care Tips

- Avoid synthetic fragrances. Although they're imperfect and incomplete, product labels can be helpful. Read them, and if you see the word "fragrance" in the list of ingredients, look for a healthier alternative.

- Pay special attention to laundry products. Be aware that fragranced detergents and dryer sheets affect the items on which they were used for a very, very long time.

- As you switch to healthier, fragrance-free items, try to avoid frustration if the changes don't immediately make your home, your car, or your clothing tolerable for someone with chemical sensitivities. Time and persistence are your allies.

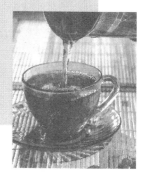

HEALTHY HOMES

The home environment is the one over which people have the most control and is an important place to make as toxin-free as possible. Numerous products contribute to the air quality in a home or other building, but they can generally be categorized, with some overlap, as those used *in* the building (such as for personal care, hobbies, furnishings, and heating), those used *on* the building (such as cleaning supplies and pest control), and those that are part *of* the building itself.

Making a home or other building truly healthy can seem overwhelming, but no step taken in that direction is a wasted step. Small steps can make a difference and can sometimes lead to enough demonstrable changes to motivate larger changes that are more difficult to implement. It may not seem possible or practical to make all the changes suggested to an existing home or building, but it's helpful to at least know some basic air quality principles in order to make safer choices in the future, when renovating an existing building, or buying or building a new one.

For those already suffering obvious effects from chemical exposures, it's wise to make changes as soon as possible, no matter how inconvenient it seems. A body can't easily repair itself while suffering continual assaults. The more quickly people are able to remove the sources of those assaults, the more likely it is that the body will heal.

The issue of keeping a home free from contaminants isn't a new one. In the Old Testament, God gave the Israelites detailed instructions on how to proceed when they found mildew (mold) in a house. The instructions included scraping walls and removing affected stones, then tearing down the house if the mildew continued to spread.[87] It was obviously not a frivolous or inconsequential matter.

When addressing the issue of safer indoor environments, healthy house experts recommend following a simple formula: eliminate, isolate, and ventilate. Eliminate toxic products. If semi-problematic products are necessary because no safer alternatives exist, isolate them completely from the breathable air. Finally, provide enough ventilation to remove or dilute pollutants that enter.

Pesticides. Knowing what to eliminate in step one is a large part of making an environment healthy. We've already touched on some of the items used *in* a home or other building that people should avoid. Of the items typically used *on* a home, those with the highest potential for harm are generally pesticides. In the informal polls I mentioned earlier, in which many chemical illness sufferers identified dryer sheets as the one item they would ban if they could, pesticides was the other most common answer. Like dryer sheets, pesticides are extremely persistent. A University of Illinois study found that no amount of washing will clean undiluted pesticide off clothes.[88] None of us on our own has the power to ban the sale of toxic products like pesticides, but we who own homes may at least have the power to ban them from our personal spaces.

Unlike the term "fragrance," the term "pesticide" does seem to carry a negative connotation for many of us. The problem is that we may not consider all the products that fall into the category in those terms, so part of the sifting process involves learning to identify those items. Is a product designed to kill something? If so, it's probably a pesticide.

Pesticide products can target bugs (such as sprays, bug bombs, mothballs, flea collars, and lice shampoo), weeds (such as weed killer and weed control fertilizer products), or even bacteria (such as antimicrobial soaps or treated clothing). Obviously, some pesticides are more harmful than others, but the potential for life-altering consequences is large enough that I urge everyone to stop and research alternatives before using any product designed to kill. A quick internet search or a trip to the library will often yield a natural solution to the pest problem that is not only magnitudes safer and surprisingly effective, but cheaper as well. The resources listed in the back of this book provide a place to start. Pesticides of all sorts have ruined and even taken lives, and I urge people to take the issue very seriously.

Cleaning products. Cleaning products are another common source of pollutants used both on and in a home or other building. They are also one of the many areas in which marketing has triumphed over common sense. Do we need a different product to clean each surface in our home or other building? Does coating something with toxic chemicals really make it clean? Kaylee notes:

> Looking back, it's hard to believe I really thought I needed all those chemicals to clean my house. I can't believe I bought into all that, and I can't believe all the money I spent!

The cheapest and safest cleaning products aren't actual products but natural materials. Water is, of course, the most basic cleaning aid. It's known as the universal solvent because of its ability to dissolve more materials than any other substance. You can enhance the power of pure water with such things as heat (a steam cleaner, for instance), pressure (a pressure washer), time (soaking an item), or special applicators such as microfiber cloths.

Water alone can't clean everything, but it can clean more than we're likely to give it credit for.

Sometimes the goal is simply to make a surface free of visible dirt. Other times the goal is to disinfect. Surprisingly, water can do that too. A test of various disinfectant products used to clean a computer keyboard found that "all disinfectants, *as well as the sterile water control,* were effective at removing or inactivating more than 95 percent of the test bacteria."[89] In other words, wiping for five seconds with clean water was as effective as wiping for five seconds with bleach, alcohol, or the other disinfectant wipes tested.

Another study of disinfectants also verified the power of water (salt water in this case) to disinfect. Researchers at the University of Alberta looked at whether a quick swipe with an antibacterial product was enough to disinfect a surface. They found that it was not and that three passes was the optimal number. Interestingly, they also found that three wipes with a saltwater solution were equally effective. The authors note, "When the surface was swiped three or more times, the saline wipe appeared to be equally effective as disinfectant wipes."[90]

Another way to disinfect is to use two spray bottles—one filled with 3 percent hydrogen peroxide (the kind commonly sold at the drugstore) and one filled with grain or apple cider vinegar. Studies show that spraying one and then the other on food or surfaces such as countertops kills virtually all salmonella, shigella, or E. coli bacteria. Researchers found the spray combination, in either order, was "more effective at killing these potentially lethal bacteria than chlorine bleach or any commercially available kitchen cleaner."[91]

The library and internet are full of natural nontoxic cleaning tips and recipes. Some of the materials most often mentioned for cleaning use are vinegar, baking soda, lemon juice, and olive oil. Other minerals and plant-based substances are also useful.

Sometimes people think that using natural and homemade cleaners is likely to be time-consuming or complicated. Annie Berthold-Bond, the author of *Clean and Green* and other books on healthier housekeeping, says:

> I have discovered that cleaning with natural materials takes
> on a simplicity similar to that of the three canisters many
> people have on their kitchen counters containing flour, sug-

ar and tea. One might instead have canisters of baking soda, washing soda, and borax, which can become as integral a part of one's life as the food canisters. Just like in making a cake, if you use the right ingredients at the right time, you have a successful result."[92]

Some natural cleaners work better than others in a given situation depending on such factors as the hardness of the water, or whether previously used products coat a surface. If one recipe doesn't work to your satisfaction, try another. It really is possible to clean in a safe, nontoxic way and to remove contaminants from your home rather than to add them.

Although most cleaning recipes are nontoxic and helpful, there are a few things to look for in them. Sometimes a recipe will include a commercial item (such as a particular brand of soap or toothpaste) as an ingredient. Obviously, the final product will be no less toxic than the ingredients included, so make sure all ingredients are, indeed, safe.

Many recipes also include essential oils. Their use is a divisive issue in the chemical illness community. Enough people find them problematic that I think it's wise to limit their use in situations where others might be exposed. If you do choose to use them, make sure they're actually essential oils rather than synthetic "fragrance" oils that sometimes masquerade as the real thing, and be sure they've been steam distilled or cold pressed rather than extracted with solvents.

Sometimes people, for whatever reason, just aren't willing to use products like vinegar and baking soda for cleaning purposes. Fortunately, safer commercial cleaners are becoming more widely available. The Environmental Working Group is a good source for information on product safety. They maintain a website and mobile app in which they give products a grade from A to F.[93]

Carpet. For an indoor environment to be truly healthy for occupants and visitors, carpet should be avoided, although it may seem more difficult to eliminate than some other products. A major carpet manufacturer told immunologist Jack Thrasher that there were "at least a thousand" chemicals used in synthetic carpeting.[94] One of the most ironic examples of new carpet sickening workers occurred when the Environmental Protection Agency renovated its office building. Employees began complaining of dizziness, headaches, rashes, breathing difficulties, nausea, and fatigue, and several workers developed full-blown chemical illness. The symptoms were blamed on a chemical that off-gassed from the carpet's latex backing.[95]

Unfortunately, carpets don't generally get a lot safer as they age. A study found that mice died when exposed to carpet samples that were as many as twelve years old.[96] As time passes, VOC levels tend to drop, but other problems develop as carpets absorb pollutants from the environment and shoes bring in chemicals from other places. In fact, environmental engineer John Roberts found that a typical carpet contains such high levels of toxic chemicals that it would trigger an environmental cleanup if found outdoors.[97]

One thing carpets collect is dust, which comes from products inside the house and contains their pollutants. A study of seventy houses in seven states found household dust to contain thirty-five toxic industrial chemicals known to cause reproductive, respiratory, and other health problems.[98] Unfortunately, Roberts didn't find vacuuming to make the carpets healthier, but actually to deposit more dust than it picked up. He reported that a house with bare floors has about one-tenth of the dust found in a house with wall-to-wall carpet. According to an article on the study, Roberts' findings suggest that pollutants in carpets could be one of the major causes of the rise in children's asthma, allergies, and cancer.[99]

Some of the most problematic chemicals found in carpet are those discussed in a previous section—pesticides. Robert Lewis of the Environmental Protection Agency examined carpets between ten and thirty-three years old and discovered that it was common to find up to five pesticides in a carpet at concentrations many times the amount generally applied in a single application. Pesticides persist for years indoors because the indoor environment protects them from the sun and rain, which degrade them.[100] Many pesticides commonly found indoors have only been approved for outdoor use.[101]

Andrew notes:

> Removing the carpets in our house made a big difference
> for me. We had hardwood floors underneath. It would have
> been worth doing even if we only had subfloor, though.

Fortunately, there are many alternatives to carpet. Ceramic tile or polished concrete are some of the healthiest flooring options. Hardwood floors can also be a very good choice, but the installation method is important (glues can be toxic) as is the choice of underlayment, finish, or sealer. Installing prefinished flooring is better for the air quality in a building than is staining and sealing a floor after it's already in place. In the flooring world, as in the world at large, it's important to be aware of misleading terminology. Laminate floors are often labeled "hardwood," and vinyl floors are often called linoleum, which is an entirely different and much more natural product.

"Heavy duty" flooring designed for commercial applications can be especially problematic. Dan Allen was the football coach at the college of the Holy Cross. He was active in the Fellowship of Christian Athletes and had founded chapters of the organization at two schools.[102] A sudden, rapid decline in his health was attributed to solvents used in redoing the gymnasium floor. Allen said, "Here I am, supposed to be this macho football coach. I was invincible, right? Nothing was going to happen to me. And the scary thing is, it could happen to anybody."[103] Coach Allen lost his fight with toxic illness, dying at the age of forty-eight and leaving a wife and three children behind.

Formaldehyde. A chemical that's quite problematic, but ubiquitous in the indoor environment, is formaldehyde. Common sources of formaldehyde are pressed wood products, such as medium density fiberboard (MDF), particleboard, or plywood, which are generally held together with glue containing urea-formaldehyde resins.[104] Kitchen cabinets are often made of pressed wood and can emit large amounts of formaldehyde as can furniture that contains particleboard (and may be misleadingly labeled as "solid wood"). True solid wood, metal, and glass are safer materials to use for cabinetry and furnishings. Although the best course of action is to avoid particleboard in the home, if it's already there and you can't immediately remove it, a specially designed sealer can improve air quality (see resource section).

Other common sources of formaldehyde in a home or other building are carpet, vinyl, foam, and fabric finishes such as on window treatments, bedding, and upholstered furniture. A smart practice when buying curtains, sheets, and other items made of fabric is never to buy anything that isn't washable and to wash, wash, wash the items (with nontoxic laundry products) and then wash them some more. Buying untreated and organic fabrics is also a great choice, of course. Formaldehyde is noted to be "a potent sensitizer" and people should avoid it as much as possible.[105]

Paints, stains, and sealers. Traditional paints, stains, and sealers can cause many health problems. Fortunately, it's much easier to find low and no-VOC paints, stains, and sealers than it once was. Unfortunately, a low-VOC product can still have problematic ingredients, but it's usually a better choice than one with higher levels of volatile organic compounds. "No-VOC" is yet another misleading term since Environmental Protection Agency regulations allow paint with less than five grams of VOC per liter to use that designation.

A general rule of thumb is that water-based paints, stains, and sealers tend to be healthier than similar oil-based products. Natural products, such as milk paint, mineral-tinted clay-based paints or plaster, and those using plant dyes are available (see resource section). There are also simple, natural options for staining wood such as using coffee or tea.

Combustion contamination. When considering factors that affect a building's indoor air quality, it's very important not to overlook methods used to heat air, water, and food. In particular, consider very carefully any combustion inside a building (burning fuels like natural gas, propane, butane, oil, coal, or wood).

Combustion produces many pollutants, the most well-known of which is carbon monoxide. When a hydrocarbon fuel burns, each carbon atom should join with two atoms of oxygen and produce carbon dioxide ("di" meaning "two"). However, when oxygen levels are insufficient, carbon will join with one oxygen atom instead and produce carbon monoxide ("mono" meaning "one").

Carbon monoxide can cause serious health problems. High levels can lead to convulsions or death, but low levels can cause symptoms that sufferers might not connect to exposure. One study found that nearly 24 percent of people who thought they had the flu were actually suffering low-level carbon monoxide poisoning.[106] One toxic illness sufferer notes:

> When we got rid of the gas in our house, it seemed like everyone in the family got more healthy, not just me.

Carbon dioxide isn't as dangerous to human health as carbon monoxide is, but elevated levels can be harmful in a number of ways. A study reported in the journal *Environmental Health Perspectives* associated indoor carbon dioxide levels with impaired decision-making.[107] Carbon dioxide can build up even in buildings without combustion sources because it's a product of human respiration. The buildup of carbon dioxide is one reason that adequate ventilation of a building is essential.

The problem with combustion isn't just by-products. Any pollutant that comes in with a fuel source (such as mold or pesticide residues on a piece of wood) becomes part of the mix.

Burning wood is problematic in other ways as well. In his book *The Healthy House*, John Bower notes that "there are over 200 pollutants in wood smoke, whose names are not easily recognized, some of which are carcinogenic." He adds that one study found that 84 percent of children in wood-heated homes experienced at least one severe symptom of acute respiratory illness during the heating season compared to only 3 percent in other homes.[108]

Common combustion sources within the home include stoves, furnaces, water heaters, dryers, and fireplaces. Attached garages can also be problematic and allow fumes from vehicles to enter the living space. Installing a ventilation fan in the garage is a very good idea. I once had a dream that I entered a house and found a car parked in the living room. I remember feeling appalled, but later I realized that homes with attached garages that don't separate exhaust fumes well from the rest of the house are probably pretty similar in their effects. Smoking cigarettes or cigars inside a home can also contribute to indoor air problems, of course.

If there are combustion sources in a building, it's vital to make sure they're well maintained and well vented. For a gas stove, that means using an overhead range hood that vents to the outside rather than relying on the ductless type that simply passes the chemical-laden air through a small filter before returning it to the room. Although essential, venting of combustion sources doesn't solve the air quality problems they create. California's Lawrence Berkeley Laboratory found that carbon monoxide and nitrogen dioxide levels from a vented natural gas stove can become as high as those in Los Angeles during a smog attack. In an unvented room, the levels can rise to three times that amount.[109] The healthiest option, and the only one for most with serious toxic illness, is not to have fuel-burning sources inside a building at all.

Many people believe that combustion appliances are cheaper to operate than electric, but this may or may not be true. Electricity and fuel prices vary widely by location and fluctuate throughout the year. Electric appliances are also much more energy efficient than they once were. One website listing the pros and cons of electric heat pumps notes, "In most areas, electricity rates are lower than natural gas, meaning that a heat pump system will cost less to operate than a gas fired furnace."[110] Although cost matters, it's a secondary issue compared to the issue of human health. Homes and other buildings with combustion appliances are also more likely to burn or explode and may cost more to insure.

Mold. Although it isn't a synthetic chemical, indoor mold can cause significant health effects as well and can contribute to the development of chemical illness. Many factors contribute to mold growth, and a proper treatment of the subject would require a separate book. It's important to control moisture (leaks, condensation, etc.) and to keep the humidity level low enough that mold can't grow. Most experts recommend keeping the humidity level below 50 percent.

There are many keys to controlling moisture and humidity. Attention to outdoor landscaping and to diverting rainwater away from the building is important. Localized ventilation fans can be very helpful installed in high-moisture areas such as kitchens, bathrooms, and laundry rooms, and dehumidifiers, either whole-house models or stand-alone units, can significantly deter mold growth. One isolated area of high humidity can cause mold to grow and then spread throughout the house or building through the ductwork or simply through natural airflow.

Bedrooms. Although most people have far more control over the air quality in their homes than they do over that in public buildings such as offices, schools, or churches, an entire overhaul of a house or apartment often feels like too much to tackle. Instead, the *Sift* stage generally begins with replacing or tossing out obviously fragranced personal care products and switching to healthier cleaners. When taking the next step, some good, often-given advice is to begin by cleaning up one room of the house (generally a bedroom), so that there's a safe place to serve as a retreat while improving the rest of the environment.

Logan instructs someone newly diagnosed.

> I started with making the bedroom a safe spot. For me this meant using glass in place of plastic, getting rid of houseplants, keeping books and printed matter out of the bedroom, getting rid of clutter. We kid around if something really bothers me and say, "Off with its head," and out it goes. Find out what bothers you most, get rid of that, then find out what still bothers you, get rid of that and soon you will have a safer area.

A mother whose son had behavioral issues shares her story.

> The most dramatic change in my son came when I took the particleboard furniture out of his bedroom. It was amazing. I would never have dreamed that just changing the bedroom furniture could pretty much give me a new kid, but it did.

The bed itself is a very important factor to consider. Conventional mattresses can be full of chemicals the sleeper inhales all night. Preston writes about the first morning she awoke after sleeping on a new, 100 percent organic cotton, flame-retardant-free mattress.

> I was free of pain. Since I had become disabled [five years earlier], pain had been my daily companion. I can't begin to describe the sense of joy and euphoria that I felt. From that day on, pain has been intermittent. Pain is no longer my constant companion![111]

Some healthy house experts advise having nothing in the bedroom but a safe bed and bedding. Not everyone is willing to be that draconian, but the general principle is to lighten the body's detoxification burden however possible, and since most people are in their bedrooms for at least eight hours or so out of every twenty-four-hour period, focusing on the toxins in that room makes sense.

This book doesn't address the topic of electromagneticfields (EMFs) in detail, but it's an important subject that may have significant implications for human health. Many experts suggest turning off the breaker to the bedroom at night and removing nonessential electrical items (replacing an electric clock with a battery-operated one, for example.) I know a number of people who've obtained relief from chronic insomnia by following that advice.

Ventilation. Because of toxins inside homes and other buildings, and because occupants consume some of the oxygen inside and replace it with carbon dioxide, it's important not to overlook the "ventilate" part of the healthy building formula. To be healthy, all buildings should provide a way for fresh air to enter and stale air to leave. I often enter an indoor space and immediately feel like an insect placed into a sealed jar without air holes punched in the lid. We know not to do that to insects, but don't seem to know not to do that to people. Lack of ventilation not only limits the amount of oxygen available, but it traps contaminants inside. It contributes to the fact that levels of many pollutants are consistently higher indoors than out. In fact, one study found that indoor air was up to seventy times more polluted than outdoor air, even in heavily contaminated areas like Los Angeles.[112]

The benefits of ventilation were more widely known in earlier years. Sanatoriums treated people with fresh air, keeping them outdoors as much as possible and the windows wide open at all times.[113] A study of army trainees found that the incidence of colds and flu was at least 45 percent higher for those housed in new barracks than for those in older buildings, a finding attributed to the lack of ventilation in the newer units. Lawson notes that "the study did not pinpoint any chemical cause, though it seems likely that what was being recirculated was a soup of alien chemicals and that the trainees in the tight buildings experienced a form of environmental illness."[114]

There are various ways to provide for ventilation. The simplest is to open windows and doors. A friend's doctor recommends opening windows for at least fifteen minutes every day, regardless of the weather. Running fans (either freestanding or ceiling fans) can help circulate the incoming air. Another simple fan-based system for freshening the air involves installing upgraded bathroom ventilation fans along with simple through-the-wall inlets in other parts of the house, often bedrooms. Whole-house ventilation systems, sometimes called air-to-air exchangers, which use ductwork (often incorporated into an existing central air and heating system), are an effective way to get fresh air into most areas of a home and provide for filtering the incoming airstream.

As in the area of combustion appliances, many people hesitate to make ventilation-related changes to their homes or other buildings because of the fear of higher utility bills. It's true that bringing in fresh air that needs heating or cooling does have an associated cost. Bower points out, however, that "the cost of tempering incoming air isn't as high as many people believe. In moderate climates it is actually quite low." He notes that in many parts of the US. the operating costs associated with mechanical ventilation are less than $100 per year.[115] To reduce costs, one can use a heat-recovery ventilator, which transfers heat from the outgoing air to the fresh air entering the building.

Even those who aren't overly concerned with the cost of ventilation may have received the cultural message that keeping a house tight, so that no air can enter or escape, is what we should do to care for the environment. Caring for the environment is, of course, a very worthy goal, but in today's context, it seems to have a limited and focused meaning. It seems to refer to protecting forests, rivers, oceans, and animals, but not to apply to the environment in which most of us spend the majority of our time. It's important that we come to see ourselves, our homes, and the air we breathe every day as part of the earth's environment, and to work to safeguard all forms of created life including human. Reducing power consumption is positive, but not when it comes at the expense of health. Our societal goal should be to produce energy cleanly and from renewable sources—not to make saving it a higher goal than saving the humans who use it.

When it comes to ventilation, the bottom line is not how much it costs or how much electricity it uses (not as much as people seem to think, in either case), but whether the benefits are worth it. That question is easy to answer. Water, food, and oxygen are necessary to human life. We simply must have fresh air to breathe in order for our bodies to function properly, and some sort of adequate ventilation of indoor spaces is a necessity. Bower notes that "the cost of ventilation should be considered just as basic as a house's foundation, walls, or cabinets. . . . We would never consider building a house without a bathtub simply because they cost money. Nor should we build a house without a ventilation system."[116] Eliminate, isolate, and don't forget to ventilate.

Air purifiers. Air purifiers can be helpful for improving indoor air quality, but they aren't a substitute for sifting through contaminants and removing as many as possible. There are a number of different types of air purifiers, each with its pros and cons, and it's important to understand that different purifiers remove different types of pollutants.

HEPA-type filters are best for removing particulate matter such as dust mites, bacteria, fungi, pet dander, and pollen. Removing gases often requires activated charcoal or zeolite filters. Some air purifiers don't have a filter at all but rely on ionization, electrostatic precipitation, or ultraviolet light. Ozone generators are sometimes marketed as air purifiers. Although ozone can be useful for cleaning up contaminants when used carefully and properly, it shouldn't be continually produced in indoor environments where people congregate.

In addition to installing freestanding air purifiers, people can improve air quality by upgrading the filter on a central air conditioning or heating unit. Filters are available to remove both particulates and gases. It's important to change the filter regularly and make sure it isn't impeding airflow.

Vigilance. Unfortunately, cleaning chemical and biological toxins from the home environment is sometimes a bit like bailing water from a leaky boat. Toxins are constantly entering, and the sifting process is never complete. Jenna, new to the world of toxic illness, wrote:

> Last week my kiddos finished some chalk art projects and I let their teacher keep them to spray with hair spray for keeping the chalk stable. My husband brought them home yesterday afternoon, and the minute he walked into the house, my head started to hurt. It took me a couple of minutes to key in that it was the pictures and they *really* smelled bad. I took them to the garage and placed them in a safe place. I still have the headache. *Grrrrr*—the lessons I have learned this year!

For those who are homebound with chemical illness, a common problem is that any family members who are out "in the world" can come home with synthetic fragrances or other chemicals clinging to clothing, skin, or hair. Some severe chemical illness sufferers require anyone entering the home (even other family members) to immediately shower and change clothes before entering the main living area. Family members are sometimes willing to do that, but it's not so easy to ask that of a repair or delivery person. For those reasons, dealing with people who enter the home is a constant source of challenge for the chemically ill as the following experience illustrates:

> I order all my supplements by mail. Usually the delivery guy leaves packages on the bench outside my door, but every now and then he rings the doorbell, and I have to open the door and be sickened by his fragrances in order to get the products that are supposed to be making me better. It's such a Catch-22. At least he doesn't come inside. A repairman was here recently, and I was sick for a week.

Mail is often a problem for those with toxic illness. The petroleum-based inks used in magazines, newspapers, and advertising flyers can cause symptoms, and magazines often contain scented perfume samples that can contaminate other items. Brett complains:

> I wish I could figure out how to donate to ministries without getting on their mailing lists. The message seems to be, "We appreciate your donation, and to thank you we're going to bombard you weekly with mailings that make you sick."

Those who don't yet have obvious health issues from chemicals don't have the same warning system that those with toxic illness do, so keeping a home's air as clean as possible means being consciously aware of the issue and learning to recognize and consider the toxicity factor of everyday items. It requires a new way of thinking. When purchasing any new product, the wise consumer will consider health ramifications even before such issues as esthetic factors and price. Sifting is a way of life for the chemically ill, and those who are currently healthy would be wise to develop the habit.

Take Care Tips

- Begin to think of the items used in, on, and for your home in terms of their human health effects. Remember the formula: eliminate, isolate, ventilate.

- Consider starting with one room and making it as toxin-free as possible then making further changes from there.

- Offer to help chemical illness sufferers with health-related home renovations that are challenging for them to do such as removing carpet or applying sealers.

CHAPTER FOUR

$\mathscr{S}$eparate

You have been called to live in freedom, my brothers and sisters.
But don't use your freedom to satisfy your sinful nature.
Instead, use your freedom to serve one another in love.
For the whole law can be summed up in this one command:
"Love your neighbor as yourself."
—Galatians 5:13–14

The phase of sifting through products and making a home environment safe is vitally important. It's a prudent measure for everyone to take, and for people who are only mildly chemically reactive, it may lower the toxic body burden enough to enable normal functioning in society. Those more seriously affected by chemicals, though, soon find that sifting through their own products is only part of what they need to do. The *Separate* phase is the stage of avoiding toxins and separating from them wherever found.

COMMUNITY CONCERNS

Perhaps the most frustrating part of the *Separate* phase is realizing that establishing and maintaining a healthy home environment is not entirely within your own control. The actions of neighbors greatly affect air quality in and around a home. This is especially true for those who live in apartments, but it's true for those who live in detached single-family homes as well.

Lawn chemicals used by neighbors can cause much suffering. A newsletter I receive noted that of thirty-four of the most common lawn chemicals, 59 percent are neurotoxic, 38 percent cause kidney or liver damage, 35 percent cause birth defects, 29 percent cause cancer, and 21 percent interfere with reproduction. In addition, a full 85 percent are sensitizers.[117] Healthy people who don't wish to develop toxic illness should pay special attention to chemicals that are sensitizers. Trading health for a yard free of weeds (plants that have fallen out of favor but pose no real danger to anyone) isn't a good bargain.

Some people don't chemically treat their lawns, but almost everyone cleans their clothes, and the choice of laundry products can greatly affect others as they're pumped directly into the neighborhood through dryer vents. Toxic illness sufferers sometimes try to learn their neighbors' habits and plan when they can take a walk or open a window around the times when they think their neighbors will be doing laundry. Researchers analyzed emissions from residential dryer vents and found more than 25 VOCs emitted. Seven of the chemicals are classified as hazardous air pollutants and two as carcinogenic with no safe exposure level.[118]

Of course, the actions of neighbors affect the chemically ill in many other ways as well. Experiences such as the following are common.

> Neighbors are putting on a new roof. I spent *all* day yesterday in the car at the local county college parking lot. Last night I came home to sleep. Smelly room but made it through.

Actions of neighbors can be literally life threatening as in the sad story of two infants, part of a set of triplets, who died after inhaling fumes from pesticides applied in a neighboring apartment. The babies' father remarked, "We never expected the cause of death to be . . . pesticides sprayed in an apartment in front of ours. We didn't even smell it from how dizzy it made us."[119]

The actions of neighbors can be life threatening in other ways too. Nancy Noren was a chemical illness sufferer who was extremely reactive to pesticides. When neighbors would use lawn chemicals, she would shut her doors and windows as quickly as possible and then flee her house. Campgrounds were a problem because of chemicals such as charcoal lighter fluid and restroom cleaning products, so she would often camp out in a remote location. That practice may have kept her safe from pesticides, but it didn't keep her safe from other dangers. Her body was found where she often fled and a young man who had noted her patterns was arrested for her murder.[120]

Take Care Tip

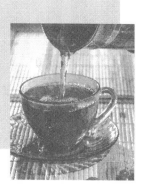

- Remember how interconnected the human family is. Think about the products you use and actions you take in terms of others living nearby.

THE WORKING WORLD

Although keeping the home environment toxin-free is a challenging job, the challenges pale in comparison to those faced in many work environments. Dr. Pamela Gibson surveyed working MCS sufferers and found that only about one fifth were working in conditions they considered safe.[121] Some environments are obviously worse than others. A study found that workers in the perfume industry, for example, were among the groups with the highest incidence rates of occupational asthma.[122] A Swedish study found a higher incidence of violent crime by painters than by all other workers,[123] and an expert reports that the average construction worker has a life expectancy ten to twelve years less than the average,[124] a fact that may well be related to their work's toxic products.

Office jobs may seem safer, but they can have plenty of their own hazards as these toxic illness sufferers can attest.

> I had to quit my state job because they would not ask another employee in the office to stop wearing perfume

that caused me to have asthma attacks every day. I am on disability now and miss my job a lot sometimes. I tried everything to stay—doctor after doctor and taking medications. Finally, I had a major meltdown in my office, and my supervisor sent me home. I knew then I couldn't go on.

———————

Of course, we know that the effects of exposures can last a long time so I never feel like I can fully recover. When I read about MCSers becoming badly incapacitated because they continued to work in an unhealthy environment, I am afraid that it will happen to me too.

———————

Once I got diagnosed, my employer still wouldn't do anything to help me out like remove perfumed air fresheners. They told me I didn't quality under the ADA. They were so wrong. They told me to accept the situation or find someone who would accommodate me. So I quit. They were in shock. They didn't think I would do it after being there eight years. I didn't either, but God had given me the strength.

Job safety laws exist, but enforcement is weak. One public health expert noted that within the same period of time, more than 125 people had been sentenced under environmental laws to more than a thousand collective years in jail, but only two employers had been prosecuted under job safety laws. They received a total sentence of forty-five days of jail time. The government spends sixty times as much protecting the environment as it does protecting workers.[125] It shouldn't be necessary to ignore either in order to protect the other.

Toxins in the workplace are dangerous for all. Johnson notes a study in which even workers who claimed to have no symptoms from chemicals in their work environment showed a decreased level of mental functioning when exposed.[126] For the more seriously affected, the ability to make a living and provide for themselves and their families may hinge on seemingly small choices made by coworkers such as whether to use fragranced products, or the choice of cleaning supplies.

It isn't at all uncommon for a chemically ill worker to raise issues of air quality in the workplace, for coworkers to take requests to change products as a personal affront and violation of rights, and for an amazing amount of animosity to grow. The depth of feeling sometimes exhibited by those asked to make changes lends some credence to the theory that sometimes people may be actually physically addicted to the chemical products they use.[127]

Linda, a nurse profiled in *Casualties of Progress*, shares about reading emails written by coworkers regarding the requests she and a few others made for a perfume-free workplace.

> I find it hard to describe my emotions when I read the email messages. I felt like I had been kicked in the stomach. After I recovered from the original shock, I started to cry. Reading how my coworkers conspired to wear heavy amounts of perfume, all the same kind on the same day, was horrifying. They even named the day according to the perfume they chose to wear that day; . . . They bragged about spraying the bathroom that we used with perfume and about spraying the top of the stairway that we used. They joked how all of us should dress up as "bubble people" for Halloween and they should dress up as cleaning products. One of the worst perfume offenders wrote on the email, "Like I said before, shoot [them]. I know where we can get some bullets."[128]

At some point, the majority of toxic illness sufferers give up the fight to stay employed in a conventional workplace. The Gibson study found only 23 percent of MCS respondents were working outside the home.[129] Most try to hold onto jobs as long as they possibly can, and generally longer than is wise. Long-timers in every chemical illness support group urge the newly affected not to make the same mistake they did and to quit work before they irreparably damage their health.

For business owners, there's a practical as well as a moral aspect to making the work environment safe. A businessman with an existing facility he was outgrowing decided to experiment by renovating an adjacent building using only nontoxic materials and pest-control methods. The buildings were of the same size, were used in the same manner, and had similar employee populations. For his efforts, the owner was rewarded with a 40 percent reduction in absenteeism for workers in the new facility.[130] A healthy building led to healthy workers and higher productivity. Christians should take the topic of toxic products seriously, simply because we represent Christ and have been told to care for our bodies and for our fellow travelers, but there are obviously financial and business benefits to addressing the issues, as well.

Take Care Tips

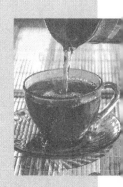

- Be aware that decisions you make about personal care and other products affect those who share your work environment.

- Don't minimize or doubt the problems others have with certain chemicals even if you don't seem to have problems with them yourself.

- Try not to take it personally if people react to chemicals on your body or clothes. Remember that they don't want to separate from you, only from the toxins that make them very ill.

- Be aware that becoming "safe" for someone with chemical sensitivities generally involves a learning process on both sides. It's likely to take time as well as a large measure of trial and error. Patience and persistence are key.

LEARNING LESSONS

Those who don't spend their days at home or work generally spend their days at school. Preschools, grade schools, middle schools, high schools, and colleges all tend to have similar air quality problems, but the youngest students may show the effects most readily. In an ABC news report, Dr. Phillip Landigan of Mount Sinai School of Medicine laments that schools use too many chemicals that no one has tested for their possible impact on young children. He adds that "children live down on the floor. They crawl on the rug. They're constantly putting their little fingers in their mouths. And all of those actions increase the child's exposure."

To test how quickly toxins might affect children at school, a team entered a classroom and applied a nontoxic powder only visible under ultraviolet light to areas where pesticides are most likely to be sprayed or settle. They then let the kids play for twenty minutes, and after that time, using UV light, they found traces of the powder all over the children's clothes, hands, and faces. The report notes that kids spend nearly 90 percent of their time indoors, yet there are no specific federal requirements limiting the use of toxins, such as pesticides, in schools.[131] The problem is far-reaching. New York's attorney general's office found that 87 percent of schools in the state used pesticides.[132]

Toxins in schools, including building, maintenance, and cleaning supplies, fragranced personal care products, and teaching materials (dry erase markers, glues, and paints for example), all contribute to filling the finite "rain barrel" that is a person's ability to detoxify chemicals. Preston writes about her school years.

> The difficulty I had concentrating and focusing on what the teacher was teaching continued all throughout my schooling. My ability to concentrate and retain the information taught fluctuated and my school marks displayed the effects. . . . Now, in hindsight, I can trace a very definite pattern linked to chemical exposures. When I had a lot of chemical exposures, my school marks were low (in the 40s, 50s, and 60s), and when I had less chemical exposures, my school marks were higher (achieving the 70s, 80s, and 90s).[133]

School is a special challenge for those who are already chemically ill like the writer of the following:

> I started a different college and managed to make it through one semester but was so sick every day when I got home that I had to crawl up the stairs. Mom started taking me to and from school, and I made it through, often taking notes with my head lying on my desk. That summer I thought I was getting better. I managed to stay mostly away from toxins. When I started school in the fall, it was in a new building. I made it through two days, but on the third, I had to leave. I had known the first time that I went in the building that I couldn't tolerate it, but I was determined not to quit. I finally realized that I had no choice if I wanted to live.

Unfortunately, the chemically ill young lady who related that experience didn't live many years longer. She lost the fight with chemicals while still very young, leaving a great deal of potential unreached.

The death of a child is probably every parent's worst nightmare, but it's not the only nightmare parents of chemically ill children face. It's common for parents to face problems with those in authority when they're assertive about their children's needs or their children miss more school than is deemed acceptable. Sometimes there are accusations of parental child abuse or neglect and threats of removing children from the home.

It's easy for the uninformed to jump to wrong conclusions. A newspaper article profiled a chemically ill child, and, after it appeared, a stranger to the family went to the school to present the administrators with an article on Munchausen by Proxy, a syndrome in which parents deliberately hurt their children in order to get attention from medical workers.[134] Donohoe shares the story of parents visited by government authorities and urges us to contemplate their situation: "Become those parents for just a moment. . . . Feel what utter powerlessness is like. What do you feel? What would you be prepared to do? How would you respond?"[135] Perhaps an even more important question is this: how can the rest of us help those parents and children and keep others from ending up in their position?

Unfortunately, the antagonism that can arise around the issue of environmental problems doesn't stop at the door to the school, but it affects educational institutions as easily as other parts of society. Donohoe tells of being contacted by a mother whose son developed neurological problems after moving to a classroom in a new section of his school. Other students in the classroom had problems as well. Although the school board was "less than enthusiastic" about an investigation of the room's air quality, they conditionally agreed. Testing the room revealed unsafe levels of several pesticides.

Dr. Donohoe drafted a report and offered to meet with the school board. The response was a refusal to meet and a threat of legal action if the doctor communicated his concern to parents. He picks up the story.

> They attempted to discredit me, despite the fact that I was the only published researcher in the field of low dose exposure risk. They held closed meetings and attacked me publicly, knowing that I could not respond because of their lawyer's threat. Drama and misinformation was everywhere . . . . Parents who felt there was a possible risk and that I should put this case to the parents, were themselves threatened with legal action if they promulgated such a view. Information flow became controlled by the school with the distribution of telephone numbers of "acceptable" authorities which the parents should telephone for reassurance. None of the experts had seen a single sick child from the school. Somewhere along the line, they forgot the children. They forgot what the consequences were if they were wrong.[136]

Take Care Tips

- If you have children in school, work with teachers, staff, and other parents to improve the school environment. If you don't have school-aged children, lend your support to those involved with the issue and encourage others to take their concerns seriously.

- Be aware that time and budget constraints are real and that schools aren't likely to become less toxic without a lot of focused education about the issue and persistence from those advocating change. Consider offering to spearhead fundraising efforts to help secure needed funds.

- Try to avoid antagonism but remember what's at stake.

SHOPPING SHOCKS

Creating a safe home is daunting, and a safe school or work environment even more so, but even if one obtains that, the hurdle of acquiring life's physical necessities, i.e., shopping, still remains. Any single toxic product inside a store can contaminate the air in the entire place. Even health food stores often carry synthetically scented products or use toxic pesticides. Shopping "surprises" like the following are constant.

> I'm so tired right now it's hard to type. I needed to do the grocery shopping today, as I had not been for a couple of weeks. At the store, I reached out to get some broccoli just as the misters came on. Got some of the water on my hands. I kept thinking that the store was more smelly than

usual. Then I realized that the smell was on my hands. They must put something in that water, which makes me wonder how much good buying organic produce there is doing me.

When I came home, I tried to wash it off with warm water and safe soap, but the smell would not come off. I called hubby for suggestions, as my brain wasn't working too well by that time. He suggested vinegar. Now my hands smell like scented vinegar.

Of course, a large problem with shopping is simply finding tolerable items to purchase. Manufacturers have decided it's a good idea to add scents to all sorts of things that many with toxic illness might otherwise find tolerable like trash bags and toilet paper. Formulas are constantly changing, so a product that was safe to buy last week might not be safe to buy today.

Even paying for items can be challenging, particularly when using cash. Bills often pick up fragrance and other chemical contamination from previous owners. The chemically ill try various things to avoid the problem including wrapping bills in aluminum foil or keeping them in the freezer until right before a shopping trip. One friend tried the following.

I slipped baking soda into my wallet to help neutralize the fragrances that always cling to the bills, but later I stopped as I wondered if some thought it was illegal drugs—this powdery substance.

Shopping online or through catalogues solves some problems but causes others. Shipping costs add up quickly, and without viewing the item, it's impossible to know what you're actually purchasing. Of course, when you buy online you can't smell the items either. I recently bought a shirt from an auction site that was advertised as new—not pre-worn and presumably not prewashed—but it arrived reeking of dryer sheet fumes. Friends have had auction items (even non-clothing items such as books) arrive with dryer sheets actually packed inside the box with them.

Shopping has always been challenging for the chemically ill but has gotten even more difficult as scent marketing (sometimes called olfactory marketing) has become increasingly common. Marketing companies offer point-of-sale services with fragranced air in the immediate vicinity of an in-store product display, or they fill an entire store with a specialized scent that the shopper can associate with the brand. One scent marketing company speaks on its website of the "Proustian Effect," which is "what happens in your brain when a smell unleashes a flood of memories."[137] Perhaps "Machiavellian," in the sense of using cunning and duplicity to achieve an end, would be a better term.

A discerning friend once pointed out that synthetic fragrances are essentially attempts to deceive us. Certain combinations of chemicals may vaguely smell like lavender, vanilla, or lemon, for example, but they have entirely different effects on us than the actual substances do, and the deception keeps us from protecting ourselves. My friend noted that Satan is the great deceiver[138] and that counterfeiting God's work is one of his favorite tools. I remember sitting on my deck one windy day and noticing that I was receiving a lovely natural aroma of flowers from one direction, but that when the wind shifted, an artificial floral scent wafting from a neighbor's dryer vent bombarded me. I remember thinking that at one time I might have found both scents pleasant, but that now they didn't even seem remotely similar. The contrast seemed very clear—God's beautiful creation on one side and the artificial (and dangerous) substitute on the other.

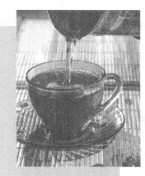

Take Care Tips

- If you're healthy and able, consider offering to help the chemically ill to do their shopping. Before making a trip to the store, ask if there are things you can pick up for them.

- If you run a shop or other business, make it as toxin-free as possible, both for your own sake and for the sake of others who enter.

Doctoring Dangers

"Shopping" for services, such as setting up utilities and bank accounts, is just as difficult as shopping for physical products. Shopping for healthcare—visiting a doctor's office—can be especially frustrating. Healthcare facilities can be as toxic as other public spaces and are sometimes worse. The shame isn't only that healthcare workers should know better, but that they evidently often do to some extent but don't put the knowledge into practice. Several doctors and nurses have told me that their training covered the importance of not wearing fragranced products around patients, but that they've never worked anywhere that enforced that policy.

I recently communicated with someone whose wife died of complications related to cancer. He noted that the actual cause of her death was chemical illness because if she hadn't been chemically ill she could have sought medical treatment as soon as the cancerous lump appeared. It's difficult to overstate the problem of toxic healthcare facilities and of workers who don't acknowledge and accommodate chemical illness.

A sufferer puts the frustration into words.

> How do you even get a broken bone set or have a regular physical when you have MCS? In some ways, it feels like a death sentence. Even if I could afford medical care, which I can't, it wouldn't matter. Entering most doctors' offices when I'm stronger than usual is enough to put me down. Entering when I'm already sick would probably put me over the edge.

Take Care Tips

- When you visit a doctor's office, clinic, or hospital, be especially attentive to synthetic fragrances and other chemicals on your body and clothes. Remember that others who are also attempting to access medical care may be in very fragile condition.

- Consider accompanying people who are chemically ill to the doctor's office or hospital to assist them. It's helpful, for example, for a healthy person to wait in the waiting room while the chemically ill patient remains outside or in the car until time for the actual appointment.

- If you work in a healthcare facility, take the responsibility seriously to make it a safe place for all. Educate, advocate, and don't give up. See the resource section for helpful materials.

The Trouble with Travel

Working, shopping, and visiting friends are challenging activities for those with toxic illness, and traveling can be even more so. Even short trips around town can be difficult, since the interiors of buses, taxis, subways, and cars are often toxic environments. The challenge of public transportation includes sharing the air with others using fragranced and otherwise toxic products, but even riding in your own car alone can be a risky undertaking.

A report entitled "Toxic at Any Speed: Chemicals in Cars & the Need for Safe Alternatives," looked at two classes of toxic compounds. It revealed that concentrations of some toxic chemicals in automobile interiors were five to ten times higher than those found in most homes and offices, which are not exactly healthy places themselves. The researchers found associations between the chemicals examined and neuro-developmental damage, thyroid hormone disruption, birth defects, impaired learning, liver toxicity, premature births, and early puberty among other health problems.[139]

Finding a tolerable car is often a huge problem for people with chemical illness. Finding a used car that has off-gassed many of the "new car" chemicals but hasn't accumulated other chemical contamination is a bit like looking for the proverbial needle in a haystack. Generally, cars are cleaned with toxic products, have air "fresheners" used in them, or pick up fragrances from users' bodies or clothes. The detailing process used by most car dealers can make any detailed vehicle, even an otherwise tolerable one, unusable for the seriously chemically ill. I have chemically ill friends I've known for over a decade now who've been looking for a safe-for-them vehicle the entire time I've known them.

Getting around town can be a challenge, but longer trips can seem almost impossible. Hotels are full of hazards and airplane flight can be disastrous. Airplanes, of course, share the hazards common to other public spaces, but they have their own special issues. Janine Ridings, founder of the Aroma of Christ ministry to the chemically ill and author of *Comfort in the Storm*, tells of a life-altering airplane flight. She writes, "As we neared our destination . . . my so far perfect flight turned into an MCS sufferer's nightmare. We hit a severe storm, which resulted in three aborted landing attempts. After each failed attempt, the plane shot back up into the air, each time allowing toxic fumes that smelled like jet fuel to enter the cabin through the ventilation system.[140]

Her experience may not be an isolated one. A CNN report notes that the air inside an airplane cabin is half recirculated air and half "bleed air," which bleeds off the engines and that "if an engine oil seal leaks, aviation engineers and scientists say, the bleed air can become contaminated with toxins." The report adds that individual factors, such as taking certain medications, may make you more sensitive to the effects of the fumes.[141]

For the chemically ill, even traveling in a safe car and staying in the home of a friend or family member is an adventure full of potential problems as the following story illustrates:

We stayed at a hotel on the way to our son's house, and I thought I did okay. The next day, however, I had a terrible headache. I eventually got some relief before entering my son's house that he assured me was scent-proofed before I came. A strong fragrance hit me when I walked in the door, and my tongue started getting thick, and breathing was difficult. My husband went into action and found a scented candle on the table as part of a centerpiece. I also found a scented bath and body soap in the bathroom (these are everywhere it seems). My husband put these in the laundry room and shut the door. I was glad my daughter-in-law wasn't home yet when we got there, and my son was fine with moving the things. I went immediately to our bedroom that had been stripped of bedding and put the sheets, blankets, and pillows I brought with me on the bed. Even though my husband had opened windows while I was in the bedroom, I still got a lot of exposure to fragrances and was miserable most of that night.

A challenging road trip. Traveling is a rare and risky proposition for me as it is for most with serious toxic illness. I no longer stay in hotels, but I used to occasionally attempt it on rare occasions in the summer. When the weather was warm enough, I could leave the room windows open and sleep in the car if the room proved unworkable. The last time I attempted it was on a trip I took because it was cheap (I accompanied my late husband as he attended a work-related conference) and because I was completely desperate to escape my house. We communicated with the hotel staff to find the best option, and many things about the accommodations seemed promising. The building was older, hadn't been recently renovated, and had windows I could open. We reserved a room at the end of a hall, near an outside entrance, so I didn't need to walk through a toxin-filled lobby to get in and out. The bottom line, though, was that it was a public place (a Christian conference center) used by the general population with all their conventional products.

When we arrived late at night, the strong odor of fragranced cleaning products greeted us instantly. The main problem seemed to be the bathroom, so we put our air filter in there, shut the door, and pointed a box fan at it to try to keep the fumes contained. Next, we stripped the bed of the hotel linens and put on our own. The pillow was very fragrant (it had undoubtedly picked up contamination from people's hair products), so I also switched that for one of mine from home. I settled down to try to sleep but realized the mattress pad was also a problem, so we removed that and remade the bed. I attempted sleep again, but my nose led me this time to the blanket. We removed the blanket, and my long-suffering husband went out to the car to bring in a sleeping bag to use as a blanket instead. That modification allowed me to sleep for a few hours, but I woke up again in increasing pain and still reacting to synthetic fragrances.

At this point, I had two guesses about the problem. The first was that the cleaning products used in the bathroom were affecting me. The second possibility was that the mattress itself was contaminated. I didn't know what else to do about the bathroom, so I decided to try to put more layers between the mattress and myself. I zipped up the sleeping bag, so I could sleep in it on top of the bedding. This did improve the situation, but it didn't eliminate all exposures from the mattress (which I could now tell was, indeed, a source of fragrance residue). The next morning we stripped the bed again and flipped the mattress over. I also put a towel between the mattress and the bottom sheet. My pain level continued to rise to the point that I decided to sleep in the car for the rest of the trip and use the hotel room only for brief forays in and out.

Once I had decided how to sleep, the next problem was to figure out how to eat. Because of extensive food allergies and the difficulties of eating in public places like restaurants or conference dining halls, I always travel with all my food precooked and frozen. When we made room reservations months earlier, we also reserved a small refrigerator. Unfortunately, when we arrived we were told that all were in use and none were currently available. After a day or two, the staff was able to procure a refrigerator that was missing parts (it had no shelves), but it kept my food edible, and I was grateful for it.

The problems of eating and sleeping were now solved. The next problem to solve was how to work. I was pleased to find that I could run an extension cord out the hotel window so I could use my laptop computer while I sat outside. Because my husband had a preconference meeting to attend before the main session, the hotel was fairly empty the first day or two. I was happy to be able to sit outside and have the place essentially to myself. It worked pretty well—until I glanced up at one point and saw a very large black bear coming my direction! He was close and coming closer, and since the door to the hotel was between us, I had to go toward him (while he stared at me) to get inside. It was a rather scary experience.

Despite the bear encounter, I decided to risk using the spot again the next day. Unfortunately, the location was no longer usable for other reasons. Cleaning product fumes wafted from the open windows all day long. Once the hotel began to fill with conference attendees, personal care product fumes wafted from the windows as well.

I never did solve the problem of how to work for any length of time on the computer because I never found an electrical outlet I could use in a clean-air environment. I tried using a nice covered porch with an outdoor outlet, but it was near open windows, which caused the same problems I had behind my hotel. I started sitting in the car, trying to use the computer as long as possible before the battery died, but that proved problematic too. At one point a man next to me in the parking lot decided to put oil in his car, and I couldn't go anywhere to escape because on a trip into town the day before to refill my oxygen tanks, we ran over some nails and developed two flat tires. The situation reminded me again of the basic toxic illness truth that in general, our ability to function is in the hands of strangers. This is what it means to have chemical illness. This is what it means to try to separate from toxins.

Take Care Tips

- Be aware that products you use in hotel rooms and other public lodging will affect those who come behind you. Do your part to keep them as toxin-free as possible.

- Keep your car as chemical-free as you are able and consider selling it privately rather than through a dealer who will 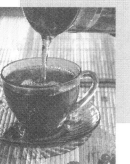 detail it and likely make it less usable for someone with chemical illness. When you sell, consider advertising your car as chemically safer, which will aid those looking for vehicles tolerable for them.

THE MOVE TO MASKS

Chemical illness sufferers in the *Separate* stage gradually become aware of how truly pervasive synthetic fragrances and other toxic products are in our environment. Once they understand that fact, they often try to attack the problem by wearing some sort of mask. Chris says:

> I never thought that I would need a mask. I knew I was going to get better as I was just going to avoid perfume like my doctor said. Ha, I had no idea of all the items that had the same chemicals in them.

Wearing a mask in public involves clearing an emotional hurdle. The illness goes from invisible to visible, and wearers become targets of stares, remarks, and all sorts of strange reactions. Riley's reaction to needing a mask is typical.

> I'm embarrassed to wear my mask so I tell myself, "It's not

that bad" and sometimes go into a store without it and suffer for days after.

People treat you differently when you're wearing a mask. Fear is a common reaction. Once a little girl stared at me then said to her mother, "I'm scared. Let's go home." People often move away, which can be a good thing if they're wearing fragranced products. My husband once explained to someone why I was wearing a mask, and the person then remarked to me, "Well, I'm glad that's the reason, and you're not wearing it because you have a disease I might catch from you." It's obvious that people are often afraid of that scenario, but I had never had someone voice that thought aloud to me before. In a way, I admired his honesty, but I wasn't sure how to respond.

Wearing a mask also poses logistical challenges like this one.

> At church, I usually wear a charcoal mask. I have yet to figure out how to wear it to the church dinners and still be able to eat.

Eating is impossible in a mask, and conversing can be very difficult as well. The masked person is able to watch and listen to the activity but is essentially unable to participate. The biggest problem with masks, however, is that they don't work very well, as found in a study by Millqvist and Lowhagen and verified by toxic illness sufferers everywhere.[142] The study found that perfume provocation (with a nasal clamp used to prevent patients from knowing if they were breathing perfume or a placebo) could provoke patient symptoms and that breathing through a carbon filter mask had no protective effect. Masks didn't solve the problem for the following people, either.

> I am able to attend church now but only for the hour service if I wear my mask. The children stared at me a lot, but I talked to them and let them know it was me, and I was wearing the mask because I was sick right now. It took a lot of courage to walk in that door because I am basically a shy person who doesn't like a lot of attention on me, but I was

determined to worship God no matter what others think. Afterward I was exhausted and had to take oxygen.

———◦———

How I hate this disease! MCS is getting more and more difficult to cope with. Last weekend I was feeling good so I decided to risk going to a church I know has mold (bad idea). I thought if I wore my mask, I would make it through okay. It was so good to see the members I had not seen in weeks and hear a wonderful sermon. I seemed to be doing fine. I could smell the mold through my mask but it was not overwhelming, and I coughed some but didn't start wheezing. After the service, I had to go directly outside because I was feeling faint. Outside, I took off my mask and tried to take a big breath of fresh air but could not get any in. My daughter followed me out (thank God). She said, "Mom, your face is really red. Where is your inhaler?" I couldn't speak and was wheezing uncontrollably. I just handed her my purse and she got my inhaler and handed it to me. I'm beginning to fear I might not make it through one of these attacks. It's getting scary.

It's common for the chemically ill to progress from cloth masks to half-face or full-face respirators. These work for some, but others find it difficult to breathe in them or they find themselves sensitive to their materials. Some use powered respirators, as used in industrial settings, but must deal with the weight, the noise, and the price of the replacement filters even if they're able to tolerate the materials.

Even the industrial-type masks and respirators must match the chemicals in the environment. Two workers in Chicago died after inhaling fumes from a product they were using to strip wax from a bathroom floor. A spokesperson from the Occupational Safety and Health Administration said the masks they were given were inadequate for use with a particular chemical in the product.[143]

In addition to protecting themselves with masks, chemically ill people often find that covering the body is also important. Diane has a respirator and cover-up she uses when she leaves the house that she thinks makes her look like Darth Vader.

> A neighbor took me to the store to return something my daughter bought. The customer service woman *never* looked at me, asked me why I was returning the item, asked for my credit card, or by any word acknowledged that I was there. I know I look strange in my "Darth Vader" cover-up, but I usually get stared at, not ignored. It's a new experience to be invisible. Normally when I am in public it is amazing how many cell phones are pointed in my direction. I wonder if pictures of my "Darth Vader" cover-up have made it around the world yet?

Personally, I once counted over twenty masks and respirators in my possession. Although I found some to provide a measure of help, none of them have ever given me the freedom I seek. Some people (including me) find using supplemental oxygen helpful, but it requires a prescription, and insurance generally doesn't cover it for the chemically ill, so the cost can make its use prohibitive.

Masks are not only inconvenient and seldom fully effective. A very serious drawback to masks is that in many places they're actually illegal. There are many horror stories of suspicious police stopping toxic illness suffers in masks who then have to endure hours of exposures and questioning while attempting to prove they don't have hostile intentions. I've heard of people in masks getting stopped and questioned in places you might expect, such as on a bench in front of a bank, and in places where you wouldn't, such as simply driving down the street.

The chemically ill teenager who relates the following story got off easier than some.

> Last night my mom and I were coming back from a doctor's appointment trip, and the car needed gas. With my MCS, I can't be in the car when my mom is fueling up without

getting a huge reaction that affects my airways. So my mom dropped me off at a park, which was down the street from the gas station.

So I am waiting for my mom, wearing my mask, and a police car drives up. Two policemen come out of the car and ask me what I am doing. I told them that my mom was down the street getting gas and that I have MCS and can't handle the fumes. One of the policemen says, "Right," with the tone of "Yeah, right"—he didn't believe me.

Of course, they had fragrance on them, so I was reacting, and my lungs were burning, and I was having a hard time breathing. So I told them that I was about to step back because I was reacting to their laundry soap. And the policeman says again, "Right" in the same tone as before, so I stepped back, and they stepped forward.

Then he asked if I was from around the area and if I had ID. About then my mom pulled up. She runs out of the car yelling, "If you have cologne on, you are causing her damage" and telling them all that I had told them before.

Then they allowed me to go, and I got in the car and put on my oxygen and took all the detox agents that I had. Let me just say, my legs were trembling, and I was scared. Getting approached by police is scary, especially when you aren't doing anything wrong.

I have my own gas station and mask story. After my husband died, I needed to somehow manage the tasks he did for us including buying groceries and gassing up the car. My first attempt to put gas in the car myself involved wearing my mask. The mask didn't keep all the fumes from me, and I knew I was going to pay a price, but I was still congratulating myself for managing to get through the ordeal more or less successfully when I pulled out of the station, mask still on my face.

I had gone less than half a block when a sheriff's car pulled out behind me. At first, I thought nothing of it, but at some point, I realized the car was making every turn I did. I live on a dead-end road, and the route to my house from the gas station includes other dead-end roads. It's not a well-traveled path. The vehicle followed me all the way home until I pulled into my driveway, and it continued down the street. Maybe it was a coincidence, or maybe my mask made me look suspicious. I'm a middle-aged white woman. If I were in a demographic more likely to be profiled, I would be extremely wary of wearing a mask, no matter how much I needed it.

Take Care Tips

- If you see someone wearing a respirator or mask, don't assume they have a contagious disease or have just come from robbing a bank. Smile, but if wearing scented products, don't get too close.

- Do what you can to make public spaces healthy enough that masks or respirators won't be needed.

The Challenge of Church

For chemically ill Christians, one of the hardest places to separate from chemicals is the church environment. Problems, as with other buildings, tend to include the building materials themselves, a lack of adequate ventilation, cleaning products, methods of heating, lawn care products, and pest control methods. Churches are sometimes worse than other places, though, because those who enter the building bring many toxins with them. People tend to put on more perfume when coming to church and sometimes wear clothes that have been recently dry-cleaned. Some churches and faith traditions also routinely use scented candles or synthetic incense.

Despite the fact that they tend to be very toxic places, attending church is generally one of the last activities that Christians with chemical illness are willing to give up. They fight hard to keep going, well after the point at which problems are obvious, as the following experiences illustrate:

> I always react to some degree in church: sometimes a little, sometimes a lot, but I try to sit quietly (suppressing my coughs) and endure as much as I can. Church and fellowship are such hard issues for those of us with MCS. Because I really don't like to attract attention, I run to my car after church and cough and breathe and recuperate until I feel well enough to drive home.

> Well, I know I'm repeating "old news" when I say churches can be some of the worst places for MCS persons to enter. This frustration has been stated more times than I can remember. I have personally known persons that have had reactions in churches bad enough they were transported to the ER for, say, a full-blown asthma attack triggered when someone got next to them highly scented. It can be a true medical emergency to some.

Sometimes a church situation that was once tolerable will become unmanageable as the chemically ill person's condition changes. For example:

> When we moved here, we started attending a small church. The sanctuary area was not very good for me, but I was hopeful that I could educate people. Since the church is struggling to grow, I hoped they might feel it was worth working to help me. I did get some good responses. Some people really avoided wearing products. The pastor even started opening a couple of outside doors for a while the day before the services to air out the building (which was unused most of the week). But last year I had a bad cigarette smoke exposure and became more sensitive to secondhand smoke. I realized that some people in the church

were smokers and even though they didn't smoke at church (although occasionally they would smoke right outside the church), the smoke on people's clothing and hair was a problem for me. So for the past year or so I haven't been going to church. We've tried a few other churches in the area, but I react to just being in the building, so it seems pointless to try to get people to wear less "product."

Often, it's not the physical condition of toxic illness sufferers that changes, but the toxins used inside the church building.

I had a hard time at church. My heart started racing, and I couldn't sing a note as I couldn't breathe well. I wish I would have left, but since I am the pastor's wife, I fight to stay as long as I can. I was told a new person is cleaning the church.

Early steps. Churchgoers with toxic illness usually don't stop attending services and activities immediately when they discover the church environment is causing them harm. A common first step is to experiment with sitting in different areas of the sanctuary in an attempt to find a pocket of clean air. Sometimes the air in front is cleaner, but getting to it involves navigating an obstacle course of perfumed parishioners, and leaving early or changing spots is hard to do unobtrusively. It's very common for the chemically ill to move from one spot to another as fellow worshipers come in and find their seats. One chemically reactive person described it as a game of musical chairs.

Another early step is to give up the activities and services deemed most toxic, an approach taken by these chemically ill Christians.

Even when I could still go to church, I didn't go on holidays. I discovered that they were the high perfume days so I avoided those. I would usually volunteer for the nursery or something else then.

It's encouraging to know that there are churches that see the need for fragrance free areas. I am not at all sure, though, that to designate an area will even begin to be enough as Sunday when I walked into the sanctuary it was SO strong and thick. I felt like I could have cut the air with a knife. When I talked to our pastor's wife this morning, I told her I would be very happy if they could simply make the children's church area safe for my son, and I would just stay down there on Sundays and help. Wednesdays there are only a handful of people, and I think I can then simply sit a ways back from most of them. At least I am going to try that.

Sitting in the back, away from the crowd, is a common coping technique for those not yet willing to give up church attendance. It is certainly an imperfect solution. The following are typical challenges:

At first, I sat away from everyone else, feeling weird and alone. I couldn't hear where I sat, so I missed most of what was being said. I would sneak in and out doors where no one else was coming and going. Sometimes nothing worked as one strongly fragranced person can ruin the air in all the room. Once my husband preached in a small church, and the three ladies that came early were enough to run me outta there. I spent the hour in the car, thankfully in warm weather.

———— ••◦•• ————

At our old church, the ladies hold an annual Ladies Retreat. From Friday night till Sunday afternoon, we enjoyed well-organized activities including Bible studies led by our pastor, having prayer pals, time alone with the Lord, all meals together, evening fun program (most of us participating), and staying in cottages, about six or eight to a cottage, all by a beautiful lake. I'd never had so much fun, or been so inspired, as when I enjoyed those retreats. Then

MCS made it all change. Just getting there was a problem as I couldn't drive that far anymore and couldn't be in a car with fragrances. Eating meals was a problem—had to sit way in back and hope no fragranced people sat at my table. Same with the Bible studies and evening fun. The last time I went, a lady who understood my problems took me in her van, I had a room alone, sat in the back for everything (where I couldn't hear), and generally felt ALL ALONE. I decided if I'm going to be lonely, I'd rather do it at home alone. I must have gone to fifteen of those, but finally it was not possible.

Giving up. Finally, it isn't possible. This is the truth that many, many people with chemical sensitivities have had to learn. At some point, the struggle becomes too much, and there don't seem to be any options left except to admit defeat as the following chemical illness sufferers finally did:

I go to Wednesday night services and sit back from the group, although I need to sit farther back as I had a definite reaction this last week. I take the kids in through the downstairs door so they don't go through where most of the cologned people are. I am not sure what it was, but my son was definitely exposed to something this Wednesday though, as Thursday morning was a bit of hell. I told my husband that we would go again this week, but if we have the same kind of day on Thursday, I am going to stay at home with him for a time. I *hate* staying home from church.

———•◦◦◦◦◦•———

I kept going to our old church then leaving fifteen minutes later. Each time I hoped it would be different. Finally, I cried all the way home and just quit going. It was SO HARD.

———•◦◦◦◦◦•———

I finally just gave up trying to go to church. I've cried buckets of tears over it, but there's not a thing I can do to change things. The church can change the situation, but I can't.

Sometimes a church will try to address a chemically ill member's spiritual needs by suggesting that the member lead a home Bible study group. This is workable for some but impractical for many. One problem is that fellow group members, unless they are unusually well educated on chemical issues, are likely to bring fragrance and other chemical residue with them into the home, no matter how much they think they are chemically "clean." The chemicals linger and affect the safety of the toxic illness sufferer's home. Another problem is that people who are chronically ill can't predict when they'll be functional and able to lead a group and when they'll be stuck in bed, unable to move. For most, committing to an every-week-at-the-same-time responsibility is very daunting and unlikely to work out well.

Avoiding chemical exposures is a great challenge, but people do it for one reason—it's the only thing that relieves their very real and very intense suffering. What appears irrational behavior to those observing it is, in fact, very rational given the circumstances, as those who have learned that explain.

> It wasn't until I started having windows of wellness and was able to be the mom and wife I desired to be, that my husband understood that it wasn't a game I was playing. He said he sees now what I do when I'm well and finally gets it that I still desire to do it when I'm not well. I'm so grateful for that transition in our marriage.

I've noticed changes as I've been able to avoid as many exposures. My mind is clearer than it has been in years, and I have way more energy than I have had for some time.

I'm so very grateful to God for showing me how to improve my health by avoiding chemicals. It's a hard way to live but is a million times better than the way I was living before.

People enter the *Sift* and *Separate* phases hoping that avoiding chemical triggers will be enough to restore health. For some, especially those in the early stages of chemical illness, it is indeed enough. Others, unfortunately, find that their toxic illness journey is only beginning.

Take Care Tips

- Work to make your church a toxin-free environment, which is accessible to all and doesn't contribute to sickening those who enter. See the resource section for materials that may be helpful.

- Help build bridges so that people who have had to "separate" can still be involved in the church community. This may involve things like providing for participation in Bible study or prayer groups by telephone or video, or by providing Sunday School materials for the chemically reactive to use at home. If you have a safe home and can educate a few others to be fragrance and toxin free, you may be able to provide a safe home Bible study/prayer group, which would be invaluable to those hungry for Christian fellowship but sensitive to chemicals.

- Provide opportunities for those cut off from church activities to participate in ministries that fit their gifts, talents, and health limitations. Present options, but don't push people to participate in projects they don't feel are a good fit for them. Ministries may include such things as calling visitors, writing notes to other shut-ins, office work that can be done from home, or videotaping a solo for playing in the worship service. Ask the homebound for their own ideas and thoughts on ways they can be involved with the church.

$\mathcal{S}$trike

Show me the right path, O Lord;
point out the road for me to follow.
—Psalm 25:4

C hemical illness sufferers find relief in isolation, but their isolation also causes them extreme difficulty both in practical and emotional ways. They want to function as normal in social and work settings and participate fully in activities they once enjoyed. They want their health back. The *Strike* stage is the stage of striking out at the illness and actively pursuing treatments of all sorts—traditional, alternative, under a doctor's supervision or no supervision at all, based on reading, word-of-mouth, studies, faith, hope, or just pure desperation.

Unlimited Options; Limited Funds

Because chemical illness is so poorly understood, there's no one standard, conventional treatment. However, fortunately or unfortunately, depending on your point of view, those who are chemically ill are never at a loss for treatments to try. Joelle describes a typical scenario.

> My husband spoke at my son's church last night sharing a testimony of how God has led us in the past. It really encouraged me and reminded me that He is with me always.

> Met a man there who sells herbal products. Wants me to attend a meeting about it tomorrow night. Says it cured him of autoimmune disease.

The phenomenon of church members offering advice and selling potential cures is extremely widespread. At the beginning of the *Strike* stage, ill people are optimistic. They believe the testimonials they hear and the promises of well-meaning, enthusiastic promoters of a particular product or treatment. It seems to me that Christians tend to be more optimistic in this stage than non-Christians are. They pray for guidance and tend to believe when they hear or read about a treatment that it's an answer to their prayers. Perhaps it is. On the other hand, hope and desperation can sometimes cloud and confuse our perceptions.

Because people in the early *Strike* stage are optimistic and believe that whatever treatment they've decided to try will restore their health, they often use up their savings or go into debt for medical care. (I was tempted to name this chapter *"Spend."*) They believe, as the following people did, that once they regain their health they'll be able to work again and replace the money lost.

> I totally relate to bankruptcy from all this. I sold my home to pay for treatments. Thought I'd get better and rebuild, and well, here I am with MCS.

———————

> After seeing my doctor and paying for my meds, I'm busted. I really need to get back to work soon before we go bankrupt, but my body is not bouncing back as well this time.

Unfortunately, the odds are very slim that the first treatment someone tries will result in significant health improvement. The odds don't seem to improve much with the second or third treatments either. The more common pattern is that sufferers try one product or treatment after another as funds dwindle away.

Environmental Health Perspectives reported on a study that examined the self-reported treatment efficacy of over a hundred treatments used by MCS sufferers. The study found that participants had consulted an average of twelve health care providers and had spent over one-third of their annual income on health care costs. In addition to the money spent on doctors and treatments, respondents had spent an average of $57,000 attempting to create safe homes.[144]

The number of health care providers seen is interesting, but it doesn't equate to the number of treatments tried, which tends to be significantly higher because of the number of over-the-counter products and programs used. Toxic illness sufferer Kim Palmer related her experiences on her website.

> I began a disheartening journey through both the traditional and alternative medical realms, seeking answers and not only receiving none but being disparaged, told it was psychological, and put on treatments that worsened my condition. After five years I figured things out from my own reading and began treatment for Candida, allergies etc., finally definitely receiving benefits though short-lived. I tried everything from desensitization shots in Texas to live cell therapy in Mexico to antiparasitics in Arizona to cavitation surgeries in Oklahoma to drops in British Columbia to diets to herbs to mega vitamins to hormone therapies to auto-urine to drugs to acupuncture to energetic desensitization to IVs to hypnosis to antifungals to homeopathy to energetic medicine to mercury removal to sauna detox to extensive testing to neuropeptides to thyroid to NAET to scar neutralizing . . . to other unmentionable therapies. In my early ignorance I even found out one traditional MD had me on experimental fertility drugs during which time I could have born quintuplets![145]

Palmer lost her fight with chemical illness. I understand that the official cause of death was "failure to thrive." As her list of therapies proves, failure to thrive doesn't equal failure to try. Peter summed up the continual search for help when, after having side effects from a supplement he said:

> So, back to square one, or, as I like to refer to it, square "-1,235,769."

Unfortunately, trying and trying to find the answer but coming up empty of solutions and funds is an extremely common pattern. The Chemical Injury Information Network receives at least one call per month from people with toxic illness who've spent all their funds trying to get well and have been promised a cure if they can just come up with "another $1,000."[146]

The situation isn't unique to our generation. The Bible tells of a woman desperate for healing. Mark 5:26 says that "she had suffered a great deal from many doctors, and over the years she had spent everything she had to pay them, but she had gotten no better. In fact, she had gotten worse." Sometimes people talk about "the Proverbs 31 woman." Frankly, I've never felt like a Proverbs 31 woman. She has far more energy than I do. The Mark 5:26 woman, though, is my soul mate. Another Mark 5:26 woman writes:

> I spent my savings. When I ran out of money, the doctor
> told me to avoid perfume. I knew that before I spent all
> that money.

In the treatment efficacy study mentioned earlier, participants had consulted an average of twelve health care providers, but they'd found only three of them helpful. And of all the treatments rated, the three that ranked the highest in "user satisfaction" were creating a chemical-free living space, chemical avoidance, and prayer.[147]

Take Care Tips

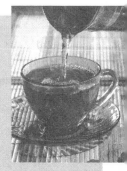

- Feel free to share information about products or procedures that have helped you or others, but understand that there may be very good reasons (a tight budget or problematic ingredients in a product, for instance) why someone will be unable to act on your suggestion.

- If you feel led to contribute monetarily toward someone's quest for health, they will undoubtedly appreciate it greatly, but be aware that there are no guarantees any given course of treatment will lead to improvement. Avoid expecting an automatic "return" on your investment.

To Doctor or Not to Doctor

There are various factors to consider when deciding what treatment options to pursue. The first question is whether to seek medical treatment at all or to assume that if God wants you to be healed that he'll heal you supernaturally, without human intervention. The question comes up from time to time in online support groups with questions and comments like these.

> I am trying to understand what my spiritual duty is as regards my healing. I am trying to understand what I should trust to him and what to science. I think that dealing with healing can be a duty to "render unto Caesar what is Caesar's." I think we have some spiritual duties to respond to the current society, not only through its laws, but its norms as well. I also believe, like Ben Franklin said, "God heals, and physicians take the credit." I am willing to go through a process for him out of obedience. But how do I know that is what he wants me to do and not a temptation of the devil. Or the reverse? That my unwillingness to go through is not the temptation from the devil?

I personally think that God gave us the ability to think, explore, and discover. Medicine is one aspect of that process. I think that God is pleased when medical knowledge is used to save lives and improve the quality of life for many.

Humble doctors will admit that while they have many tools that promote healing and good health, they are not the ones who do the actual healing. An honest look into medical history will point out many cases where treatments that should have worked didn't, and ones that shouldn't have did.

So in my opinion, when we go to doctors, we should be looking for tools, not expecting them to heal us. I think that we can make use of their knowledge and experience to help us care for our bodies. At the same time, we can maintain our faith that God is ultimately responsible for what happens to us.

There's much to say about this issue. Some Bible teachers make an interesting argument for applying medical knowledge to physical problems when discussing James 5:14. The verse says, "If you are sick, ask the church leaders to come and pray for you. Ask them to put olive oil on you in the name of the Lord" (CEV). Scholars have pointed out that there are two words for the act of applying oil. One word is "chrio," which means "to anoint." It's related to the word "Christ," which means "anointed one." The word James uses, however, is "aleipho," which means to apply or rub the oil. Evidently, the term was sometimes used when referring to massaging an athlete or applying salves and was frequently used in medical treatises. To apply oil to the body, many teachers explain, meant to use oil medicinally. The elders were to both pray and to use the "medicine" they had available.

The Bible frequently mentions medicinal plants and their associated oils or salves. In Jeremiah 8:22, the prophet asks rhetorically, "Is there no medicine in Gilead? Is there no physician there?" The question was rhetorical because the medicine of Gilead, also called the "balm of Gilead," was abundant in the region. In fact, the Israelites, after claiming the land, had a profitable trade in the expensive balm. Jeremiah was asking, "If you're sick, why not use the medicine God has given you?" In context, Jeremiah seems to be speaking metaphorically and making a spiritual point, but the question could certainly apply on the physical plane as well.

Paul's advice to Timothy to "drink a little wine for the sake of your stomach because you are sick so often"[148] was essentially a prescription to use the "medicine" available at the time. Hezekiah 20:1–7 also mentions a prescription. Hezekiah was ill and about to die. God declared that he would heal him and add fifteen years to his life. Upon hearing that word from God, the prophet Isaiah instructed Hezekiah's servants to make an ointment from figs. When they did so and used it on Hezekiah, he recovered.

I believe that, in general, we're to handle healing resources God provides in the same way we manage other resources from him. We know that food comes from God, but we take the seeds he provides and grow a garden, or we buy what someone else has grown, and then we cook the food and put it on our plate. We don't expect it to miraculously appear there or say that it would if God wanted us to eat. Even in the Old Testament when God provided manna for his people, he expected them to gather and prepare it.

Of course, God *can* heal miraculously without any human intervention, and I'm sure that's what most ill Christians earnestly desire. God's thoughts are not our thoughts, and his reasons for circumventing the laws of nature he set up are his and his alone. In general, though, I believe that most of the time God expects us to search for solutions when we're sick and be a steward of the resources he has given us.

Jesus healed in many ways. Sometimes the sick came to him, and sometimes he went to them. Sometimes he healed with a word and sometimes a touch. Jesus often reached out and touched those who needed healing, but sometimes touching him or just his cloak brought healing instead.[149] Many people begged for healing, but sometimes Jesus healed those who didn't even ask.[150]

At times casting out demons was part of Jesus's healing ministry, but often it wasn't mentioned or the two activities seemed separate.[151] Sometimes forgiveness of sins seemed part of the illness and healing picture, but sometimes Jesus specifically said that no sin was involved.[152] Some believe that his use of mud for healing the blind man[153] was, in effect, a type of medical treatment. The point is that God is both creative and personal, tailoring intervention to each person's unique circumstances and needs. He may wish to heal one toxic illness sufferer through conventional medicine, one through alternative means, and one through no medical intervention at all.

Take Care Tips

- When praying for someone reactive to chemicals, pray not only in general terms for healing, but for specific needs such as the ability to see helpful doctors with safe office buildings, for safe transportation to appointments, and for insurance coverage or other means to pay for products and services.

- Consider giving health-related birthday or Christmas gifts such as gift certificates to health food stores (assuming recipients can shop there or have someone who will do it for them) or vitamins and supplements that the toxic illness sufferer uses or has expressed a desire to try.

- If you're close to chemically ill people, consider helping them to make a list of supplements or actions to take during a chemical exposure, then remind them of the list when needed. The brain fog caused by chemical reactions sometimes causes people with toxic illness to forget what it is they need to do to help themselves when they most need the help.

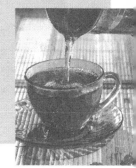

DECISIONS, DECISIONS

We'll discuss the issue of divine healing further in subsequent chapters. Let's look now at some questions we can ask when deciding what treatment options to explore.

How much money should I spend? We've already mentioned one important question. How much money should be spent on the quest for improved health? This isn't an easy question for anyone, but it becomes even more complicated for those who are married, and especially for those with children in the home. The question becomes whether spending money on health pursuits will be more positive for the family resulting in a healthy spouse or parent, or negative, with money spent on a fruitless quest for health instead of other things the family needs. If money spent guaranteed results, knowing how much to spend would be far easier, but obviously the correlation between spending and degree of health improvement is far from perfect. There's no easy answer to the question of how much to invest, but if rough percentages or general principles are in place (such as whether or not going into debt is acceptable), answering questions about specific treatments can become a bit easier.

Sometimes it's possible to save money on a therapy such as by making a home sauna rather than buying one or buying an oxygen concentrator rather than paying to refill oxygen canisters. Sometimes people save money by buying vitamins or supplements in bulk. Occasionally (very rarely for those with toxic illness), insurance will cover a helpful treatment. Obviously, it's important for spouses to share major financial decisions. Marci writes:

> One reason we had to sell our home was because we couldn't afford our house payment and medical treatment for me at the same time, so we chose to take care of me rather than keep our home. I'm thankful for a husband willing to make sacrifices to help me get medical treatment. You can always buy another home or find another place to live, but you only have one body.

What to spend on the sick family member versus the rest of the family is one "division of funds" question. Another is how much to allocate to pursue improved health versus adapting to the health you have. "Adapting" can include buying masks or respirators, wheelchairs or scooters, or even expensive chemically safe RVs or specially designed homes. Again, there are no easy answers, but if you decide on general principles or percentages, then specifics are easier to determine.

Will it work? A very basic question to answer when deciding what treatments to pursue is whether or not a product or procedure is likely to be beneficial. Unfortunately, most treatments for MCS help no more than about 25 percent of the people who try them.[154] Ultimately, the question of whether a particular treatment will work can't be fully answered without trying it, but as time passes and people gain more experience with various types of treatments and products, educated guesses are possible. It's more difficult to do at the beginning of the illness. Jordan says:

> It's so hard to know what to do. I was expected to make costly decisions when I had the least amount of knowledge or brains to do it.

In general, there's a tendency to think that "standard" medical treatments are more likely to be helpful. Unfortunately, even for people with diseases better understood than toxic illness, many medical treatments are more experimental than proven. One working group concluded that "estimates range widely concerning the proportion of medical care in the United States that is based on, or supported by, adequate evidence. However, . . . some place this figure at well below half."[155]

Many people reactive to chemicals learn quickly that they don't metabolize pharmaceutical drugs well, so a large part of trying to heal generally involves seeing alternative health practitioners or, more often, because of lack of funds, simply trying supplements and other products without much guidance. Cassidy says:

> The doctor set me on such an expensive path of treatment, I had to drop out—in fact, her bill was one that went into our bankruptcy!!! Looks like I am caught between a rock and a hard place! So I just go it alone.

Going it alone means wading through oceans of information, trying to separate truth from hype. It isn't always easy to do. Some basic questions I consider before spending money on a product are:

- **What is my guess as to the seller's motivation?** There really are some "snake oil salesmen" who see desperate people as a ripe opportunity to make money from inferior products. On the other hand, sellers may truly believe in products they sell because they've seen results both in themselves and others. The Christian faith of sellers and clients often comes into play in complicated ways. There are Christians who sell products because they believe in them and see their work as a type of ministry, and there are others who, knowing the faith of their clients, use Christianity as a selling tool. Sometimes they insinuate that the client owes them the sale because of their shared beliefs or they state that a product is sure to work because a fellow believer developed it. Sometimes motivations change through the years, and once well-meaning sellers may find themselves pushing products that aren't appropriate for every condition. Motivation isn't easy (really, not even possible) to judge, and even the noblest motivations don't guarantee a product's effectiveness or safety, of course. Some people have found good information from sales clerks at health food stores who don't make a commission or have much to gain personally by sharing the knowledge they've gleaned through the years.

• **Are there unbiased testimonials I can read somewhere?** Sometimes a company website will publish testimonials. These are interesting but hard to verify. Testimonials from unbiased sites not selling anything are worth considering more seriously. A large part of the conversation in online chemical illness support groups tends to be discussions and questions about treatments and products. Advice and testimonials from fellow chemical illness sufferers can be helpful, but of course there's no guarantee that any two people will have the same reaction to a product.

• **Can I believe the statistics cited about this product?** Where did they come from? A personal "red flag" is any treatment that claims an 85 percent success rate. For some reason, a huge number of products and treatments seem to make that claim, but I've never seen references to actual studies verifying the percentage. I've decided that 85 percent is a good number to pull from the air. It sounds impressive but not excessive. I'm tempted to claim that 85 percent of health products claim an 85 percent success rate, but I would be making that up. Undoubtedly, there are products and treatments that can legitimately claim a high degree of effectiveness, but I always view statistics with a large degree of skepticism. Percentages are tricky things. If clients don't reorder a product, it's possible for the sellers to interpret that as meaning that the first bottle proved to be a cure.

- **What are the ingredients in this product?** Are there safety concerns? It's wise to research ingredients for contraindications or possible interactions with other products. Those of us with extensive sensitivities need to look at every ingredient including fillers, dyes, preservatives, flavorings, etc. The form or source of a specific vitamin, supplement, or medication can also make a large difference in effectiveness and tolerance.

Will it make me worse? Another very important question to ask when deciding on treatments is what the likelihood is that a given product or procedure will worsen, rather than improve, the health picture. Jody notes:

> Even if we are fortunate enough to find a doctor who has lots of experience treating these illnesses and even if they seem to be compassionate and confident that they can provide results, they just don't live inside our bodies. Some doctors seem to feel that they really understand what's going on, but results show that they are still practicing a pretty "hit and miss" form of medicine at this point. We need to be very cautious about what we expose ourselves to.

Even disregarding the actual treatment, the doctor's office itself often (very often) causes problems for chemically ill patients. Very few doctors are in tune with indoor air quality issues, so even walking in the door can be problematic. Dylan's experience isn't unusual.

> My specialist left me in the room for an hour. It took three weeks to recover from that visit. Now I stand outside at my nurse practitioner's office and put my nose against the window so they don't forget me.

How do you decide how much risk to take? There are many variables to consider. Some parents become more aggressive in pursuing treatment for themselves as their children grow older and the consequences for a worsened condition aren't as great as when the children were more dependent. Sometimes people with toxic illness who are still working outside the home are less willing to take risks that might affect their ability to earn a living. It's wise for the chemically ill to consider how much risk of worsening their condition they're willing to take at any given time.

A toxic illness sufferer with years of experience shares her treatment philosophy.

- Cocoon whatever wellness I already have.

- Take "tortoise steps" to gain more wellness—a new supplement, food elimination, a little exercise, a noninvasive test, a little detox, a little therapy. Listen to my body. Pray. Negotiate for tiny steps.

- As much as possible, set up strong, compatible support systems for such things as practical help, advocacy, therapy, and safe housing.

- Maintain self-nurture and support systems at all times—to help me cope, enhance wellness, get me to another level, and help me take another tortoise step.

- When there is improvement, add on big stuff like major testing and detox.

Even when someone with toxic illness decides that a particular treatment has a low probability of improving health, the question remains whether there might be other reasons for seeing a doctor or health practitioner. Frankly, sometimes chemically ill people are so isolated and lonely that they continue to see doctors who aren't helping them much because the trip to the doctor is their only social outlet, and the emotional boost is worth the cost of the appointment. Other motives are more altruistic such as educating physicians on the realities of toxic illness and serving as a guinea pig for the benefit of those patients who'll come later. Some Christian patients find sharing Christ's love with medical staff part of their purpose. A patient who keeps in mind broad goals for seeing a doctor is less likely to succumb to depression or despair when treatments don't bring improved health.

Will it affect me spiritually? The most important question of all when deciding what healing modalities to pursue is how a certain treatment might affect a sufferer's spiritual well-being. The question of what treatments are spiritually "okay" can lead to much conflict, both internally and with other believers. I imagine the great majority of chronically ill Christians struggle with the issue, and I certainly don't claim to have definitive answers. I do, however, have some broad guidelines that I use when attempting to make these important decisions.

- **If in doubt, don't do it.** The body is temporal, but the spirit is eternal, so spiritual considerations are paramount. Continue to pray and to learn as much as possible about treatment modalities. Sometimes a treatment you're not comfortable with at one point in your life may look different later, after more prayer and study, or a course you've been pursuing will start to seem questionable. Monitor spiritual health as well as physical health. If it starts to seem more difficult to pray, for example, it's wise to evaluate everything that's changed in your life that might be contributing to that.

- **Don't let others make your decisions for you.** It's certainly wise to take the counsel of doctors, other health practitioners, friends, family, and fellow toxic illness sufferers, but in the end you're the steward of your own body and the one accountable to God for the decisions you make. The fact that a treatment did or didn't work for another, or is or isn't something others feel spiritually comfortable with, is food for thought, but it doesn't answer the question of whether it's right for you. It isn't always easy to discern his voice, but as much as possible try to discuss treatment plans with the Great Physician and not be distracted by the multitude of others giving well-intentioned advice.

- **Evaluate where the healing from any given treatment originates.** Imagine that a child—we'll call her Judy—gets a cut. Her mother puts a bandage on it that's covered in purple polka dots. The cut heals, and the mother thinks it must have been the purple polka dots that did the trick. The next time she puts on the bandage she says, "Praise the power of purple polka dots." She repeats her mantra each time she puts on the bandage and jumps up and down while turning in a circle, symbolically making polka dots on the floor. Judy's mother then buys a special purple polka-dotted shirt that she wears performing her ritual. Because Judy's cuts always heal, Judy's mother is convinced she's doing the right things.

What is the source of power that heals the cuts? Judy's mother thinks it comes from purple polka dots. The truth is that it comes from the healing powers that God put in the human body when he created us.

I believe that well-meaning Christians sometimes make the same mistake Judy's mother made. We see that treatments with ungodly elements seem to produce results so we attribute the healing power to Satan. Does Satan have power? The Bible clearly teaches that he does (although God limits it). However, the Bible also calls Satan a deceiver.[156] What would give him more pleasure than to take credit for God's work? There are opposing traps to fall into in this area. One, about which we're often warned, is that to pursue healing with satanic roots would lead to spiritual bondage. The other is to reject healing from God because Satan has tried to claim credit for it. The Pharisees fell into this trap when they accused Jesus of performing miracles through the power of Satan.[157] It's easy to back away from a ditch on one side of the road and fall into one on the other side.

- **Determine whether an "iffy" treatment has a valid element that can be separated from what doesn't glorify God.** The final question to ask relates to the previous one. Let's return to our story about Judy. As a child, Judy doesn't question her mother. Eventually, however, Judy loses her faith in purple polka dots and realizes they have no inherent power. The danger is that in rejecting the method of treating cuts that she learned growing up, Judy will fail to separate the helpful element (covering cuts with a bandage) from the unhelpful and will reject that element of the treatment along with the rest.

Christians avoid many treatment modalities because they're somehow associated with ungodly elements. The danger, however, is that, like Judy, we'll simply discard the whole package without determining if there's something at the core God wants to use.

Success in the *Strike* phase depends on many factors. When treatments match sufferers' physical imbalances (and their budgets), they can attain much health improvement. If not, sufferers move into the *Sigh* phase, where hope becomes harder to find.

Take Care Tips

- Help provide the chemically ill with the three things shown most helpful: chemical avoidance, a chemical-free living space, and prayer.

- Be aware of needs for big-ticket items such as saunas, wheelchairs, organic mattresses, and air purifiers, and help people find ways to acquire these if you can.

- Pray that those who are ill will have wisdom and discernment as they make decisions about treatments to try. Provide input if led to do so but remember that ultimately all people are stewards of their own resources and health and responsible for their own decisions.

CHAPTER SIX

Sigh

My heart is breaking as I remember how it used to be:
I walked among the crowds of worshipers,
leading a great procession to the house of God,
singing for joy and giving thanks.
—Psalm 42:4

The *Sigh* stage is the stage of impatience, depression, and grief. In the *Sift* stage, sufferers create spaces for themselves that initially seem like healing and nurturing sanctuaries. Unfortunately, they start feeling more like prisons as time goes on.

Christians often seem to enter the illness experience with a certain resignation—a sense that they need to pass through a valley in order to learn a lesson or facilitate some greater good but with confidence that they'll emerge stronger and better on the other side. The problem comes when the valley is wider, deeper, darker, and longer than ever imagined. We cling to the hope and promise of heaven but recoil from the prospect of an earthly life lived in the valley. For the chronically ill, living in the valley involves struggling to meet physical, emotional, and spiritual needs.

Physical Needs

The severity of chemical illness spans the gamut, of course, but people who are homebound because of their reactions have often had enough damage done to their bodies that they're still quite limited in daily functioning, even when isolated from as many chemical exposures as possible. The sheer amount of extra work required for a chemically ill person to provide for basic needs compounds the problem. The following toxic illness sufferers lament that fact.

> I find that most people don't seem to get why it takes us so long to do things. Sometimes I think to myself, "Something that a well person can do in an afternoon might take me a week or a month or even ten years to accomplish." For me, it's because of the cognitive dysfunction as well as the muscle weakness and the low energy. Now I'm also aging and my body systems are breaking down faster. I'm in more pain, and there are some things which have become impossible to do.

> I feel so overwhelmed by the simple things that others take for granted and the total lack of understanding of how difficult it is once disabled to accomplish these things.

> One of the problems that I face that is the most frustrating is the lack of time because eating, sleeping, and merely surviving take up so much effort and energy that little is left over.

So what *does* take so long? Consider the basic needs of food, clothing, and shelter.

Food. The Bible tells us that there's more to life than feeding ourselves,[158] but it's hard to deny that we need to regularly fuel these physical bodies.

Many who are chemically ill can't easily shop for groceries, or safely enter most restaurants, and because of food allergies or the need to eat organically, they may need to cook their food from scratch. Toxic illness sufferers with families often cook separate meals for themselves and for family members. If health permits, the chemically ill sometimes try growing their own gardens, but they may find they can't be outside when necessary because of the fumes from neighborhood dryer vents or neighbors' use of lawn chemicals. Chemicals used by neighbors can drift, contaminate the garden, and defeat the entire purpose. It's not just gardens that can become contaminated, either, as the following experiences demonstrate:

> During the Christmas season, my heavily perfumed wonderful Christian neighbor gave us some peanut butter fudge. It sat in the decorative jar for a while, and I felt guilty for not trying it so I popped a TINY piece into my mouth. I immediately realized my mistake. I could taste her perfume, so I spit it out and rinsed my mouth out, but it was too late. My mouth and throat burned, my throat swelled, I lost my voice, I got a headache, and I was sick for hours.

> It's bad enough that I have to smell the hand lotion on the clerk who checks me out at the health food store, but I'm really, really tired of tasting it on the food I buy there and having to toss so much of it out. I end up having to keep going back to the store again and again, playing the odds and hoping this time I'll end up with something I can actually eat.

Although many healthy people do all their grocery and household shopping at one place, that doesn't always work for those with toxic illness. Many people reactive to chemicals only buy food from stores that don't sell other products, such as dryer sheets, which can permeate the air and contaminate food inside the building. Even when the store environment is acceptable, food can still be contaminated. Often it becomes contaminated during the transportation process, inside a truck, for example, that recently transported something else.

Food contamination, especially by pesticide residues, is a problem for everyone. An estimated 20,000 Americans a year will develop cancer because of pesticide contamination of food they eat.[159] For the chemically ill, the issue is vitally important. However, it sometimes seems like the more one needs to eat fresh, organic, healthy food, the harder it is to either afford or acquire, as Rosie's experience illustrates.

> There's a local co-op in town where you can get organic food semi-affordably. Unfortunately, it's a "working" co-op, where you have to help set up tables, unload food from the truck, etc. Obviously, there's no way I can do that. Last year my husband and I decided to give it a try, but it's just not working. He can't give up half a day and drop everything else on his agenda whenever the truck rolls in. The co-op seems to be set up for healthy, stay-at-home moms, and if you don't fit that profile, I don't know how you're supposed to make it work.

I know of one chemically ill person who tried to get around co-op delivery problems by volunteering her house as the drop-off point, but she had to give it up because the fumes from the delivery truck sickened her.

Take Care Tips

- Be aware that personal care products you use may affect any food you handle, so if you help with church dinners, work in a grocery store, or simply share food with friends, be attentive to the need to remain as toxin-free as possible.

- If you're a gardener, avoid using chemical products on your produce, both for the sake of yourself and your family, and so that you can safely share any extra food with others.

Clothing. Chemically ill people can have an extremely difficult time finding acceptable clothing. Challenges include what they can tolerate, what they can afford, and what they can easily acquire. Some with toxic illness can tolerate synthetic fabrics, but many can't. Some have trouble with dyes. Some wear only undyed organic cotton.

Even those who can wear clothing made of a variety of fabrics have challenges related to purchasing them. Do you enter a toxic store and face being sick for days or weeks? Do you order things from a catalogue or online in the hope that they'll fit and be chemically tolerable? Some of us do the bulk of our shopping at garage sales because it's safer for us than entering toxic stores, and it more easily fits our medical-expenses-stretched budgets, but used clothing is almost always heavily contaminated with strongly fragranced, toxic laundry products.

Once a toxic illness sufferer buys something, whether new or used, the next challenge is making it safe to wear. New clothing can contain many different chemicals, including antifungals, dyes, and formaldehyde-based finishes. Used clothes are generally contaminated with detergent and fabric softener residue. Even previously tolerated clothing can be made unusable for a variety of reasons, the most common being the use of public washers and dryers. As previously noted, laundry products, especially dryer sheets, tend to coat the surfaces of the appliances and then transfer chemicals to all clothing washed in them.

Making clothing safe to wear can be an exhausting, extensive, and expensive proposition. Upton writes:

> We have finally given up with most used things. . . . We usually have to wash new things 15 to 20 times to make them tolerable for me.[160]

I've also mostly given up on used clothing, but when I used to purchase it my process for making it wearable went something like this.

- Purchase clothing at a garage sale, often wearing gloves and a mask.

- Upon returning home, turn clothing inside out (to avoid sun-bleaching issues), hang them up, and put them outside in a hidden area equipped with a hanging bar for the purpose.

- Leave items outside for months. Occasionally, when it rains, move items so they can get rained on.

- When a clothing item has aired enough that it can come in the house, bring it in and soak it for several days in vinegar.

- After a few days, begin washing the item over and over again, adding different decontamination aids to each wash as needed, such as baking soda, sodium percarbonate, or borax.

- If, after a few days of washing, the item still isn't tolerable, put it outside again and wait a few more weeks or months.

- When the item is finally tolerable, try it on. If it's too small, put it in the giveaway pile. If it's too large, put in the "try to fix" pile. Check it over closely because if it fits, it may still be unusable or need repair because of sun-bleached areas or holes that the bugs have eaten in it during its sojourn outside.

There are countless methods for trying to decontaminate clothing. One method utilizes a pressure cooker. Other creative attempts involve burying clothing in the dirt or tying an item to an object on the shore and dropping it in a fast-moving stream. Some people recommend sprinkling clothes with powdered clay or using a device containing an ultraviolet light.

The process of clothing decontamination is complicated further when the chemically reactive person is trying to buy clothing for children or other family members. It involves guessing what sizes and styles will be appropriate by the time the item will be safe to be near. Some creative souls have tried to avoid clothing problems by having clothing made of whatever safe material they can tolerate, such as tea towels or vintage tablecloths. Rita shares a success story.

> Well, my seamstress has outdone herself with my latest outfit. I gave her thirteen tea towels from the 40s or 50s because I knew that it was totally safe material for me. It took

lots of piecework to get it to fit together. She even went the extra mile and crocheted yellow lace on the bottom of the yoke and some on the neckline. It looks so feminine. She had mailed it to me, and it was like waiting for Santa to come. What a blessing she has been to me.

Take Care Tips

- Use people-safe laundry products, not only for your own health, but for the good of those who may wear the clothes after you've passed them on.

- If you use public laundry facilities, be aware of the fact that chemical residue from products used will remain in the machines and will transfer to other items washed and dried later.

- If you have a relatively toxin-free home, washer, and dryer, consider offering to let a chemically ill friend without safe laundry facilities use your machines.

- Do you sew? If so, consider using your skill to help the chemically ill acquire clothing that is safe for them to wear.

Shelter. Acquiring safe clothing is a challenging issue, but the quest for safe shelter is an even larger and sometimes overwhelming one. Lawson writes about Anni, who began sleeping on her porch to avoid cigarette smoke coming from a neighboring apartment. In order to improve her situation, she looked into 450 different houses or apartments without finding any that would work within her health and budget constraints.[161] Finding or making a safe place to live is one of the biggest issues chemically ill people face. Dr. Pamela Gibson notes that "the use of toxic materials in buildings and the ubiquitous nature of chemical exposures render most living situations unsuitable for those with MCS."[162] Statistics tell the story:

- Gibson and colleagues found that 66 percent of people with MCS had lived in unusual conditions, such as their cars, in RVs, on porches, or in tents at some time in their illness. One survey respondent reported living for a year in her horse trailer.[163]

- A study out of Massachusetts found that 57 percent of MCS sufferers had been homeless at some point, and 10 to 20 percent of respondents were homeless at the time of the survey.

- Twenty-five percent had lived in a car, for an average of nine months.

- Fifteen percent had lived in a tent, for an average of eight months.

- Seventy-three percent had at some point had to live in places that made them sick.

- Only 25 percent considered their current housing to be both safe and permanent.[164]

When I began writing this book, I was aware of the facts I just listed and of the serious housing crisis among the chemically ill. What started as intellectual understanding, however, became personal experience. A water intrusion in my basement led to an increase in the level of mold, and since my mold sensitivities are extreme, the house became unlivable for me.

At first, I was unable to be inside my house at all, so I split my time between the deck, the garage, and the thirty-year-old campervan we bought and renovated after it became clear I could no longer stay in hotels. Gradually, as we worked on the house, I was able to be inside for longer periods during the day. After five months, I was able to move back inside.

Unfortunately, my time inside was short-lived. A humid summer caused the mold levels to rise again, and once more I was forced out. I spent the next several years able to be inside the house all day without problems, but unable to sleep inside at night. I was grateful to have the campervan, but it wasn't a very comfortable bedroom when winter temperatures dropped. Upton understands that. She writes:

> Over all, I have slept in our car about five or six nights.
> Not bad considering what others go through. Other times I
> slept on decks, patios, driveways, in a shed, in the open air
> on grass, in a tent, in a camping cabin in January, or in a
> camper so cold there was ice frozen to the aluminum floor.[165]

As with so much else involving toxic illness, the epidemic of homelessness is most often hidden from view, largely because homeless shelters are not accessible to people suffering from toxic illness. Commenting on the Massachusetts report, disability activist Susan Malloy stated, "I'm furious that zero respondents have been able to stay in a homeless shelter." Noting the lack of safety inherent in MCS homelessness, she added that "practical self-defense measures should preclude the way we have to live."[166]

The lack of permanence for even those with currently safe housing is due to many factors, including the ever-changing neighborhood environment and the uncertainties of rental situations for those who don't own their residences. Problems are rife, even when property owners are compassionate and understanding. A newspaper article reported on a landlord wishing to sell a property she was currently renting to a woman with toxic illness but wanting to help her tenant find a workable and affordable place to move to before she did so. Contacting various charities didn't lead to any help, nor did contacting the tenant's church. The landlord asked, "Is there not one charitable organization, not one church in our community that could assist?"[167]

The need for affordable safe housing for those with chemical illness led to the building of Ecology House in California. The eleven units have what they describe as "a long, nationwide waiting list."[168] My understanding is that "long" means many years and that most people on the list will never make it to the top.

Searching for safe living quarters, researching neighborhoods, attempting to make an imperfect situation tolerable, moving belongings again and again—this is a common MCS life. Sometimes it becomes even more complicated than usual as it did for the following toxic illness sufferer:

> Currently I'm homeless. I've been sleeping in my car (took
> passenger seat out and put framing in for a small bed,
> quite comfortable actually), and more recently a friend has

accommodated me temporarily by making several changes in her guest room so I can be in it (sort of). We have sequestered me off. The attached bathroom has become my kitchen, with small refrigerator, electric frying pan, etc. The front door is not too far away so I can scoot in and out easily.

My husband had a tumor removed a year ago (his illness was the reason we left our safe house), and he had radioactive dye inserted. Ever since then, I can't be with him. Makes me very sick. So, our life has been full of change, right and left.

We've been looking for a home with bedrooms that are apart from one another that's safe for me. Something where he could be on one side and me on the other but have been unable to find anything I can be in, so we're reverting to what we started with years ago—taking a 1970s Airstream, gutting it, and making it environmentally safe. We are thinking of doing two (if we can afford it) so he can have one with an office for him and me the other. We are currently scouring everywhere trying to find older Airstreams for sale.

Even those with fairly toxin-free homes have the challenge of keeping them that way since all homes need maintenance. There's no such thing as a "simple" repair or renovation. Something as seemingly minor as replacing caulk can displace a chemically ill person from a house for weeks or months. Sometimes what's meant to improve a house makes it completely unlivable.

As previously noted, products used by neighbors can also make a home unsafe. The author of an article entitled "The New Homeless" writes about building a nontoxic house but finding that herbicides used in her neighborhood were entering and contaminating her home. She writes, "My husband and I now find ourselves forced to move once again. . . . We will have to live further out from family, medical care, organic groceries, just so I can try to have some quality of life."[169]

Take Care Tip

- If you need additional motivation for making your home as toxin-free as possible, consider the fact that if your home is safe, you may be able to provide temporary shelter for chemically ill friends who have to leave their homes temporarily because of such activities as neighborhood yard chemical applications or roadwork on their street.

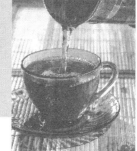

EMOTIONAL NEEDS

Physical needs are sometimes easier to see than emotional needs, but emotional needs are every bit as real. This category covers relationships, both to ourselves and to those around us.

Relationship to ourselves. A chronic illness changes people's view of who they are. Most people with toxic illness have had to give up jobs, social activities that defined them, and much more. Who have we become? Do we know ourselves? Do we like ourselves? The question of identity is one that looms large. Struggles such as the following are the norm:

> God keeps saying, "Just be" and my response is, "Be what?" Give me a task, even something like washing floors or something. It's so hard to just be.

———◆———

Please pray for me: For the help I need to put a move together financially and emotionally. For peace and identity within myself as I struggle with the vicious illness. For the wisdom to find my "place" in the world as I lose my ability to attend school.

Sometimes identity issues relate to the loss of who we thought we were. Often they are also related to the loss of who we thought we'd become. The following toxic illness sufferers had visions of themselves that chemical illness took away:

> I often don't feel like I have an important or productive role in society since I'm not working to support myself. I'm really having to come to terms with reevaluating my dreams and goals.

————•◦◦◦◦————

> The question I am trying to answer for myself is, how much of my life has been destroyed, and do I have the resources I need to rebuild? When I am honest with myself, I know that I am afraid that I will always be in this state of flux— trying to figure out what to do next, wondering if I will ever really be able to make plans for the future.

I believe the chronically ill all deal with this issue, which can surface in unexpected ways. I imagined myself a missionary until retirement; and on the parenting front, I assumed my house would be open and welcoming with kids constantly coming and going. I have wonderful sons who've always done their best to protect me from exposures and that generally meant they spent time at their friends' homes instead of inviting their friends to ours. Not long before my youngest graduated from high school, I suddenly realized that I was out of time and that image of myself as a parent was never going to become a reality.

For women especially, the parenting issue causes a great deal of pain. Not being able to attend school events or participate in family activities outside the home causes many feelings of inadequacy and failure. Those who value the parental role most highly can suffer the highest amount of distress when they feel their illness adversely affects their children.

As the old self-perceived identity changes and parts fall away, new elements take their place. Unfortunately, part of the new identity can become "Someone who makes life harder for others." Guilt for being sick, illogical as it is, is nonetheless a very real problem. These toxic illness sufferers put into words what many feel.

> I know that Jesus loves me and my life is in his hands. But I'm asking for prayer for this condition and for my feelings about it. I really want to travel for a few days near Christmas to see some of my children and my granddaughter but am afraid my MCS will cause problems for everyone.

> I'm wondering again this morning if my family would be better off without me. My sickness makes life so hard for everyone.

It's common for guilt feelings about being sick and inconveniencing others to lead the chemically ill to minimize or hide the depth of their illness. This can be a very dangerous practice. Toxic illness sufferers share their experiences of trying to tough things out, smile through the storm, and hold things together somehow.

> I babysit my wonderful baby grandson at his house one or two days a week, and although his mom and dad use some unscented products, they still have scented products in their home. They don't know how sick I really get from being there. They really do try to accommodate my illness, but it's hard to make people understand what "no fragrances" really means.

> A friend from church keeps coming over to see me. She's a really sweet, wonderful person, and she thinks she's

fragrance-free, but I get really sick every time she comes. So far, I've managed to hold it together while she's actually here, so she has no idea how sick I get. She tries so hard to be safe for me that I just can't bear telling her that it's still not enough.

Take Care Tips

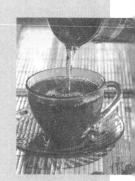

- Pray that those with chronic illnesses will be able to see themselves as God sees them and find their identity in him.

- Try to avoid words and actions that might contribute to the chemically ill feeling guilty about things they can't control.

Relationship to friends and family. Undoubtedly, maintaining healthy relationships with others is a huge challenge for people with toxic illness. To an extent, those challenges depend on whether the relationship preexisted the health decline. New relationships involve logistical challenges. Old relationships also involve grief. Grief is part of relationships on both sides of the equation because friends and family members who remember the sufferer in healthier times experience their own loss. It's no longer possible to enjoy many activities together, and sometimes those activities seem to define the relationship. Focuses and priorities have also changed, and challenges that consume the life of the chemical illness sufferer are foreign and poorly understood by healthy friends and family. Morgan notes:

> I feel like I'm failing some sort of test. I want to be accepted for how I am now, never mind what I used to be able to do.

In the *Sigh* stage, it's not just those with toxic illness who are impatient and frustrated. Friends and family members feel that way too. They may fail to understand measures that the chemically reactive take to stay healthy and misinterpret them as rejection. They don't understand the depth and breadth of symptoms and may believe that people with toxic illness are being selfish in the choices that they make. The chemically ill, on the other hand, see selfishness in others' actions and words as in the following experience:

> One of the most eye-opening moments in this whole health saga was when a friend said, "We just need to get you well so you can help me lead conferences again." Of course I want to lead conferences again, but at that moment all I could think of was, "Can't you just want me to be well because I'm suffering? Can't you want me to be well for *me*, not for *you*?" I've started to realize how conditional people's love for me really is. It's really incredibly depressing and disheartening.

Ridings speaks of trying to attend social events while navigating the attitudes of others. She writes:

> When I ask for accommodation only to see people sigh and roll their eyes at me, it makes me wish I had never bothered to ask. It makes me feel like it would be better to stay home in seclusion. People like that often feel like their party is ruined if they are not free to enjoy their scented products such as candles, potpourri, or perfume. At times when I have attended parties where the hostess has treated me with disdain, I have felt like a party wrecker. On numerous occasions, people have confessed to me that they have become physically or emotionally exhausted from trying to accommodate me. This certainly does little to brighten my day."[170]

She adds that she sometimes feels like David who wrote in Psalm 31:11–12, "I am a dread to my friends—those who see me on the street flee from me. I am forgotten by them as though I were dead. I have become like broken pottery" (NIV).

Existing relationships become challenging, but a separate challenge is how to develop new relationships after the chemically enforced isolation has begun. This challenge is particularly acute for people who move to a new area after they've become ill, but those who stay in their homes face it as well, as old friendships fall away and new ones need to take their place. How do you meet people? After you've met them, how do you maintain friendships? How do you find common activities and interests? Even a simple visit in the home, from friends new or old, can be very challenging, as the following experiences illustrate:

> It is so hard for people to remember that this never shuts off for us. A friend from church called to say that they have missed me at church lately. I have been unable to go or had to leave early because of fragrances, etc. Then she asked if I would be home Friday because she would like to stop over. I said I would, and she said, "Well, I have a perm at 10:00, so I'll probably be over about 11:00. I had to tell her that it wouldn't be possible for her to come over after she had just had a perm. It hadn't even occurred to her that this might be a problem. I have known this lady for over a year and have tried to help her understand my situation. I really do believe that she cares about me and prays for me. She just doesn't understand how prevalent the substances that make me sick are and how careful I have to be in order to avoid them. You can't compartmentalize chemical sensitivities. They are always on—just waiting to be triggered.

> A friend stopped by unexpectedly this morning. I was glad that she came, but I am not entirely sure that I should have let her stay. She had just come from a doctor's office and I could smell that strong chemical doctor's office smell on her. It's so hard to balance the need for human contact with the need for a clean environment!

Whewww!!!!!!!!!!!!!!!!!!!!!!!!! I think I *finally* got rid of the thick toxic laundry smell in my living room. Yesterday we had a couple of friends over, and unfortunately, even though they didn't wear perfume or anything, the detergent permeated *everything!* I had to scrub some of the wood chairs with vinegar. Then I had to cover my recliner with baking soda to try and soak up the fumes. I ran fans and purifiers with the windows open for several hours, and the smell *still* lingered . . . so, back to the detective drawing board. I *finally* figured out that the last culprit was the cloth tablecloth. Because the people were leaning up against the tablecloth, it reeked too. It's unbelievable how that stuff clings. The man who came over was sharing how he has developed various allergies, chronic sinusitis, etc. I hope to gently suggest they might consider changing detergents. Oh yeah, I also had to wash the two throw blankets the girl that came over used, too. If I was a healthy person, it wouldn't be so bad, but I'm exhausted from the exposure *and* having to clean up . . . this is why we *rarely* have guests over. So sad that it has to be this way.

One of the deepest emotional needs during the *Sigh* stage is for someone to understand and sympathize with the overwhelming grief for all the losses the illness brings. When I became ill, I was a missionary serving overseas, and my illness cost me my job, my identity, my home, my friends, and my adopted culture, among other things. At first, I believed that I had given up more than most MCS sufferers do. I've come to see, however, that most people with serious chemical illness give up all those things to some extent. Dr. Pamela Gibson notes, "If the effects of MCS could be summed up in three words, those words might be loss, loss, and more loss."[171]

For Christians, some of the deepest grief seems to come at the loss of a church family. Patricia shares her experience.

Belonging to a church for twenty plus years, working hard for the Lord with so many of them, coming to feel loved and appreciated by so many, they truly were my family away from home. My birth family members mostly live far away, so these folks took their place. There have been deaths in my family, both parents and my sis, but leaving a church feels like the *whole* family died all at once.

Take Care Tips

• When planning social gatherings, be aware of the needs of the chemically ill. Remember that changes made for them will make the gathering safer for everyone. Remember, too, that toxic illness sufferers did not choose to be ill and can't attend social functions without the help and cooperation of others.

• Find ways to maintain friendships with the chemically ill such as playing online games or meeting for a picnic. Be creative. Find ways to communicate that you value the person for more than just the activities you can share.

• Offer to help with child-related activities that parents with toxic illness have trouble doing. Perhaps you could attend a parent/teacher conference in the parent's place or attend a child's school performance and livestream or video-record it. The parent may also welcome help transporting children to activities.

Holding onto hope. In addition to relationship and identity losses (such as the ability to do things once enjoyed, to be independent, to exercise gifts and talents, etc.), people in the *Sigh* stage have also lost a large degree of hope. Doctors aren't helping, and accommodations by friends and coworkers aren't enough. The valley looks long and dark. The losses are extensive and very real, but they're poorly understood and rarely fully acknowledged. Most people with chemical illness walk through the valley alone.

Sometimes, even when people try to be encouraging, the message communicated has an unfortunate subtext. People often say, "I couldn't do what you do." Hopefully, they mean something like, "I'm sorry you have to live this way, and if it were me, I hope I'd handle it with grace." But instead it often seems to communicate "If I were in your place, I would kill myself."

Ridings writes that a counselor who specializes in working with chemically sensitive people says that most have thoughts about death or suicide at some point. She shares her own story.

> One day when the challenges I was facing made me question how much longer I could take the pain of life, I told my counselor, Molly, that I wanted to die. Her response to me was that I didn't really want to die—what I wanted was my circumstances to change. That made so much sense to me! When times get tough, giving up on life is not the answer. Suicide is a permanent solution to a temporary problem. The enemy loves to try and get us so discouraged that we lose hope that things will ever improve.[172]

A chemical illness sufferer profiled in *Casualties of Progress* says this:

> I never thought of suicide before I got sick. Now this thought is a constant companion. Sometimes suicide is a "rational" conjecture: I feel so [horrible], . . . I'm not getting any better—so why not? Often, however, the thought of suicide is not only irrational but unconscious. It comes not as a result of compiling all the reasons why I should, but appears ostensibly out of the blue. However, I've learned it doesn't come out of nowhere. The suicidal feeling arises when the county has sprayed herbicide alongside the road, when I'm stuck behind the diesel exhaust of a school bus, when I have the briefest close encounter with a perfumed person. Within a half hour of these and other chemical exposures, it's common that I have suicidal thoughts that are not generated by any conscious thinking process.[173]

Johnson relates the story of Abner, a chemically reactive man who testified before a Governor's Committee on the Needs of the Handicapped about the struggles of those with toxic illness, and then six weeks later took his own life. She writes that by chance she heard of three chemically ill individuals who attempted suicide within a three-week period, two of them successfully. She also noted that two toxic illness sufferers with whom she had spoken by phone during the past few years had committed suicide and another had attempted it. Johnson writes, "Time is running out for too many people with MCS. To convince them that it's worth holding on a few more months or years, it is important that society move toward an acceptance of the reality of MCS."[174]

Take Care Tips

- Help the chemically ill find hope by working to help those around you understand and acknowledge toxic illness and by doing all you can to make the world a safer place. Those who are ill have the knowledge and will, but they don't usually have the energy and strength to push for changes. People with chemical illness very much need healthy advocates.

- Don't ignore the very real physical limitations of those who are ill, but try to see beyond them. Make sure not every conversation focuses on illness. Share jokes and uplifting stories now and then.

- Sharing Christian books and other resources (audio or video) is often very welcome and can help struggling sufferers maintain hope and see beyond current circumstances. The inks may make new books and printed materials problematic, but older, well-aired books are often tolerable.

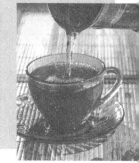

SPIRITUAL NEEDS

Physical and emotional needs are very real and extensive, but spiritual needs are the most important.

Relationship to God. The relationship to God is the most vital one in life or eternity, and the main question for the chronically ill is one Jesus asked from the cross: "Why?" "Why have you forsaken me, God?" "Why must this continue?" "Why haven't you healed me yet?" Robin shares a common experience.

> When this began, my husband and I held hands at our bed each night as we packed my neck with ice, and he prayed when I could hardly talk. All through the process we have prayed earnestly that God would guide us to the best path, the right doctors, the correct actions that would help and, in the end, glorify him. We have honestly held tight to our faith, but have been shocked beyond belief with the experiences we have had and the obvious failings time and time again with doctors, tests, and false hope. I am learning that sometimes God is silent.

So why doesn't God heal us as soon as we ask? Libraries have been written on the subject, but here are a few basics I believe and keep in mind.

- **Pain and suffering exist in the world because sin exists.** They are a consequence of the fall of humanity and an unavoidable part of life on this planet. In John 16:33, Jesus clearly says that "here on earth you will have many trials and sorrows." I don't believe a specific one-on-one relationship exists and that an individual's suffering is always tied to personal sin, but I do believe that humans are sinful creatures by nature, and we live in an imperfect, pain-filled world.

- **Sickness is one element of the pain and suffering we must endure.** Sin brought death and decay to the physical world, and our bodies are part of that world. Some argue that sickness is somehow different from all other trials and that true Christians who live by faith are immune from that particular struggle. I don't believe the Bible teaches that.

The Bible is full of examples of Christian servants who struggled with various types of illnesses. Given Paul's advice to him, Timothy must have been frequently ill.[175] In 2 Timothy 4:20, Paul plainly says that he left Trophimus sick at Miletus. Do depression and exhaustion count as being "sick"? If so, the Bible gives us the examples of Elijah and Moses, who both asked God to take their lives.[176] Job, of course, is the classic example of undeserved suffering. The Bible calls him "a man of complete integrity,"[177] but God allowed Satan to cause painful sores to cover his whole body[178], an affliction some commentators believe was leprosy. In 2 Kings 13:14, which reports on the prophet Elisha, we learn that he was "suffering from the illness from which he died" (NIV). It's difficult to claim that Elisha, whom God used to raise the dead, was a man who lacked faith.

Another "sick servant" that concisely and definitively answers the question of whether Christians can become ill is Epaphroditus. (Even his name sounds like the name of a disease: "I have arthritis, gastritis, bursitis, and Epaphroditus.") In Philippians 2:25, Paul calls him "a true brother, coworker, and fellow soldier." He also says in verse 27, "He certainly was ill; in fact, he almost died." I don't think you can argue from those verses that either Epaphroditus wasn't a servant of Christ or that he wasn't sick. He was clearly both.

When I think about the "have enough faith and you won't get sick" doctrine, I often think of the roll call of faith in Hebrews 11. That passage teaches that you can be commended for your faith and be tortured, flogged, chained, imprisoned, stoned, killed by sword, destitute, persecuted, mistreated, homeless, and sawed in two. I find it hard to reconcile the fact that those calamities can happen to Christians who are actually applauded in the Bible for their faith, but that faith will keep them from, for instance, catching a cold. What if you were stoned or sawed in two, but didn't die? Likely, you would have chronic physical symptoms. Does living with those injuries and pain, or those from flogging or other torture, count as being "sick?" If there is a distinction between "injured" and "ill," perhaps it would help to realize that toxic chemicals have indeed injured those who are chemically reactive.

- **If God healed all people, the consequences of sin in this world would be diluted, and if God healed all Christians, that would dilute and partially nullify the need for faith.** God values our faith highly and says it's of greater worth than gold.[179] When we worship God in the midst of pain, we declare our faith in God's goodness despite temporal circumstances. We express to God that we love him for who he is and not only for what he can do for us. Satan accused Job of following God simply because he made life easier. We defy Satan when we worship God in difficult circumstances.

- **God needs Christians as salt and light in all parts of his world including within the toxic illness community.** To minister to human beings, God became one. To minister to the sick and hurting, sometimes he lets those who are his hands and feet on this earth get sick and hurt too.

- **God brings order to this world with physical laws (like gravity) with specific properties of cause and effect.** Gravity keeps things from flying out into space, but it also causes people to get hurt when they jump off tall buildings. If we stay within safe boundaries (jump from a chair, but not from a building), gravity won't hurt us. Likewise, God designed our bodies to detoxify a certain amount of naturally occurring toxins. When we exceed those limits, we get symptoms that tell us that we've crossed the safe boundaries. If enough people are injured or killed jumping from tall buildings, others learn not to imitate that behavior. If enough "chemical canaries" fall ill from an overdose of synthetic toxins, surely others will take note.

- **If God always healed broken and injured bodies, none of us would die.** I remember hearing that thought from a speaker many years ago and being struck by the simple truth of it. Of course, that doesn't mean that God *never* heals. It just means he doesn't *always* heal. Sometimes it's God's will to heal us of an illness and for us to serve him in a healthy body here on earth. Sometimes it's time to exit this earthly realm, and some sort of bodily injury, sickness, or failing is the way that happens. Living forever in this fallen world in its current state isn't God's best for us. These bodies must fade away for us to receive our new ones. We should treasure and care for our bodies, but they are only temporary homes.

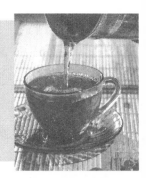

Take Care Tip

- Pray that the health challenges of those who are chronically ill won't negatively affect their faith and relationship to God.

Relationship to God's people. Some of the deepest pain for chronically ill Christians comes from feeling abandoned or forgotten by the church body. Being forgotten can manifest in various ways, one of which is in the area of prayer.

There's an understandable difference in the way people pray for acute versus chronic needs. After an injury-causing automobile accident for example, prayers of intercession flow freely for those affected, as they should. However, a year later, even if someone involved was still experiencing ill effects, it's extremely doubtful that prayers would be offered for the need at even a small fraction of the rate they were when the accident occurred. It's human nature to forget, tire of the issue, and shift the focus to other needs. The result, though, is that the longer people are ill, the less likely others are to lift them up in prayer.

I know it's difficult for those who maintain prayer lists to know when to remove someone's name. It's also extremely difficult to watch your name disappear. The chronically ill often have that experience, and Randy describes how it feels.

> I remember the feeling of complete desolation I had the
> first time I got the weekly prayer list from church, and my
> name wasn't on it anymore. It felt like everyone had written
> me off as a lost cause and completely given up on me. It's
> one of those moments that I think I'll remember the rest of
> my life.

Not long after my husband and I retired from the mission field, I went through a period of feeling unusually strong, considering all the exposures I was facing as we did what was necessary to transition to the new phase of our life. I wondered at the cause of my surprising wellness until I learned there was a rumor among my dear friends in Peru that I had been diagnosed with cancer. I realized that there was a strong possibility that my renewed health was due to focused and fervent prayer, which was, unfortunately, based on a false belief. I didn't want my friends to have wrong facts or worry unnecessarily, but part of me was honestly reluctant to correct the story. I didn't want the prayers to stop.

The truth is that prayers do stop. It's easy to forget to pray for situations that aren't continually brought to our attention, and, regrettably, it's easy to forget the people connected with those situations as well. Unfortunately, the stage in which people begin to tire of dealing with the needs of the chemically ill often coincides with the stage in which those with toxic illness find that separating from chemicals often means separating from people. This can lead to an ever-widening gulf between people who were once close and to deep feelings of loneliness and abandonment. Christians with chemical illness describe the pain of losing church relationships that once meant so much.

> I had such a hard time giving up church. I felt like a pariah
> when I stopped going. You know what shocked me most is
> that not a soul from the church called to check on me or see
> where I was. Not the pastor, not the volunteer coordinator
> whom I volunteered under, no one. I felt abandoned by the
> church, by the parishioners, by those I'd worked with for so
> many years.

I am struggling big time with the lack of response from our church in even trying to go scent free. When I don't go, I feel so much better and my child is so much more even-keeled. How do you take a child out of church, though? It has always been our social life. It's where we meet our friends, where my two kids play with theirs, etc. I have always felt it extremely important to have your children in church to hear the Word taught by someone other than Mom. I don't feel like I have much energy to fight this fight and, to be honest, if it wasn't for my kids, I would give it up in more ways than one. I don't know how to handle this. I feel like the one group of people that should be in support of what we are going through with MCS has turned their back. I have been feeling like I will explode with hurt.

I've been trying for years now to get someone from church to be a regular prayer partner and pray with me over the phone. I had absolutely no idea that it would be so hard. I know people have busy, active lives, but isn't there one person in the entire church willing to do this? Maybe I should try to get a fellow shut-in to be my prayer partner, but I really wanted to somehow be connected to the church my family attends. It's not like I'm asking for charity—this is supposed to be a two-way thing. How much should you push yourself on people who don't seem to have time for you? I've gone through plenty of hard things in my life, but I've never experienced this depth of loneliness and rejection before. I didn't expect to be so totally abandoned by God's people. There's a deep, deep, chasm in my heart.

My husband and I were very involved in our church. Even after the large worship services became too toxic for me to go on Sundays, I led Bible study, attended prayer meetings, etc. Sometimes it felt like the only day I was not at church was Sunday! However, as the church grew and my chemical sensitivities became worse, I finally reached the difficult decision that I had to stop attending all church activities. We had tried and tried and tried to get accommodation, but even the small prayer group was full of women who laughed about "forgetting" to skip their perfume. Being rejected by my church family felt almost as bad as the rejection of my needs by my parents. In some ways, it was worse because I have always understood my family dynamics, but I sincerely believed that the church cared.

I thought I was part of a church "family." I pretty much gave my life to the church, and I always believed fellow members loved me and would support me if I needed them. Now I'm rethinking everything. Did they never really care about me to begin with? Have I angered or offended people somehow? I guess what I thought was love and concern was just an illusion because you can't truly love someone and completely desert them in the time of their greatest need. I never imagined being this completely alone.

The toxic illness sufferer in the *Sigh* stage is at a point in life where spiritual connection is vitally important but very hard to obtain. The chemically ill can become extremely dry spiritually and desperate for Christian fellowship and communal worship. One sufferer heard a choir sing and said:

I'm crying all over again . . . how beautiful . . . makes me so sad for all I've lost. Reminds me of church and singing in the choir. I've been crying all day.

The desperation leads people to stand in hallways outside of sanctuaries, or even outside of church buildings, trying to hear a tiny bit of a service. It leads people to literally put their lives at risk by exposing themselves to toxins their bodies can't process. It can also lead people to attend any church or spiritual gathering at all that they can tolerate, regardless of the message or theology. Church leaders and fellow Christians, this is a serious matter. If people can't come in your building because it isn't safe for them, where will they go instead?

Take Care Tips

- Beware of the "out of sight, out of mind" tendency. Make lists or find other ways to help you remember to pray for those with ongoing needs.

- Be proactive in maintaining relationships with those out of the mainstream of society. A regular time for someone associated with the church to call and check on the homebound person can go a long way in helping the person feel less isolated and shut out. Remember the suggestions in chapter 4. It's never too late to build bridges.

CHAPTER SEVEN

Scream

There are "friends" who destroy each other,
but a real friend sticks closer than a brother.
—Proverbs 18:24

After the *Sigh* stage when the predominant emotion is grief, comes the *Scream* phase when frustration and anger become stars of the show. The circumstances are essentially the same as in the previous stage of the journey, but the response has changed. Chemical illness sufferers are no longer just grieving. They're mad.

The *Scream* phase is often very difficult, not only for those with chemical illness, but also for their friends and family members. No matter how challenging this aspect of toxic illness may be, it's difficult to get to the later stages in which hope and peace are more prevalent without first acknowledging and understanding the anger. Looking at these issues may also help friends and family members to understand why ill people may sometimes react negatively to well-meaning and seemingly innocent remarks.

LABELED

One of the things that commonly triggers anger in the chemically ill is being labeled as lazy or crazy as in the following examples:

> I've lived in this house over twenty years and have always
> been very busy till I became homebound. One day a neigh-

bor who I've always considered a friend said I had become "lazy." I just gave him a look and disappeared into my house.

I can handle trying to get my chores done. I can handle trying to somehow find my place in society, but I still cannot handle when I sense that my cousin thinks I just need to get out there and walk or volunteer or whatever. Or when my mom suggests that I might benefit from psychiatric help. I'm not crazy. I'm just unable to do what normal healthy people do in a day!

Since I can't do the family Christmas party anymore, I told a family member that I wanted to do a get together outside in the summer. My brother said that people already thought that I was crazy, and he wasn't going to do that.

The one that gets my goat is, "you are just doing this (MCS) to get attention!!!" Believe me, if I wanted attention, I would sure choose something besides isolation. Hopping on one leg would get more attention, actually.

I am getting flack from a cousin about not attending a great aunt's funeral Monday. I went last year to my cousin's funeral and stood outside. It was the loneliest feeling. I could see family inside, and I just couldn't enter that small church even with my cover-up. It would be too toxic. My cousin thinks I should just get on with my life and attend.

Marcus points out one of the dangers of these attitudes.

If I am exposed to enough doubt from others, it is actually quite dangerous. I have often allowed that doubt to make me think my health is better than it is. Then, on the basis of that false thought, I have done far more than I should have done. And I have paid a very heavy price for doing that.

Sometimes people come up with creative explanations for the "crazy" behavior they witness in chemically reactive people. A friend of mine tried hard for several years to keep somehow attending her church. She tried sitting in a "cry room" designed for mothers with small children, but it was full of the fragrances of baby products. She tried standing in the foyer, but that area was also too full of perfumes and other chemicals. Finally, she resorted to standing outside by a closed window, hearing whatever she could.

Eventually the weather and her fatigue got to be too much, and my friend gave up her attempts. When Sunday mornings rolled around, she stayed home. She tried to keep in touch with friends from church, however, and one day one of them told her something interesting. Evidently, other church members had explained her behavior by deciding she must be addicted to drugs. Her experience reminds me of the biblical Hannah who, when she was deep in prayer, was accused of being drunk.[180] The human tendency to think the worst of each other is not our most endearing quality.

Take Care Tip

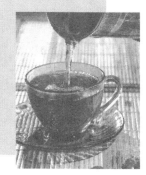

- Avoid jumping to conclusions when people's actions seem strange to you. Actions that seem irrational to observers are often very rational and sensible given the actual circumstances.

BLAMED

Another common anger trigger for those with chemical illness is the frequently-communicated message that sick people at some level choose to be ill, and if they aren't healthy, it's somehow their own fault. Sometimes people simply state that message as a fact. Often, however, people seem to believe it almost unconsciously.

Subtle messages implying that people should be able to control their own healing permeate our culture. "Get well" cards are a prime example. Sometimes a card will say, "I pray you get well soon" or "I'm hoping for quick healing," but most of the time the cards simply say, "Get well." It's an order—an imperative. The message is that healing is in your power, so do it.

Drug advertisements are another example. They tend to talk about "not surrendering to the pain" or "refusing to give in." If you're sick, you must not really be trying to get well, the message goes. You've somehow given up. Jackie notes:

> My pet peeve is a former friend who calls and says, "Aren't
> you well yet?" as though I weren't really trying hard enough.

There are various permutations of the message that people can control their own healing. One belief is that people can simply think or will themselves well. The mind is powerful, and the mysteries of the mind/body/spirit connection are fascinating and important to explore. Obviously, however, there are limits to what the mind can help the body do. People who jump from tall buildings because of drug-induced hallucinations always fall to the ground, despite their sincere belief that they can fly.

Even those most convinced of the power of the mind to heal seem to have limits to that belief. They rarely seem to expect amputated limbs to grow back, for example. Those who write books on the subject sometimes have physical limitations themselves such as the need to wear glasses. Perhaps we can control more aspects of our physical health than we currently understand, but the simple truth is that we will never be able to control everything. Omnipotence is reserved for God.

Let me be clear in saying I do believe in the wisdom and power of thinking about things that are true, honorable, right, pure, lovely, admirable, excellent, and worthy of praise, as we're urged to do in Philippians 4:8. Living life with an attitude of gratitude and a focus on joy is powerful and an important goal for us all. There are problems, though, when we don't keep this truth in balance with other biblical directives. When people instruct those with chronic illnesses to "be positive" or say, "Just don't think or talk about it," it can often feel like they are belittling or dismissing the suffering. Charlie notes:

> Somehow it seems that if you have a short-term condition it's OK to squawk about the pain and suffering, but if it's long term, you're not supposed to think about it at all, let alone mention it, or you're obsessed with it.

I once heard a preacher say the Bible says to rejoice with those who rejoice and weep with those who weep,[181] but we often act as if it says to "cheer up those who weep" instead. Of course, there are times when it's beneficial to help people remember blessings and keep an eternal perspective. First, though, people want to know that others acknowledge their suffering. This is true for all people but perhaps even more important for those whose health-mandated isolation from society makes them feel invisible.

Although many people seem to believe that all who are ill should be able to think themselves well, others acknowledge the need for outside help. A common assumption is that seeing a doctor is the simple answer to all health-related problems and that those who aren't healthy either haven't been to the doctor at all or haven't seen a specialist. Toxic illness sufferers share their frustration with that assumption.

> It's surprising how many people ask if I've seen a doctor. The assumption seems to be that I couldn't have possibly seen a doctor and still be sick. I've lost count, but I think at this point I've seen about eighteen.

My son is a paramedic. He listened to me with his stethoscope during an attack and angrily told me I needed to see another doctor—someone who could fix this. I tried to explain to him what MCS was and how it is not that easy to fix. It hurt my feelings that he was angry, but I realized that he only knows what his training has taught him and let it go. Yesterday morning he called me and apologized. He said he was really just angry at himself because he couldn't figure out my problem or help me.

Take Care Tip

• Don't state or imply to those who are ill that they could easily be healthy if they would only "think positive" or see another doctor. Trust that they very much want to be healthy and are doing everything they can to achieve that goal.

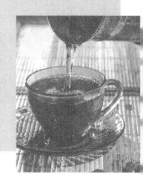

Viewed as a Problem

When people have illnesses that affect many areas of their lives, it seems common for others to begin to see them less as real multidimensional people and more as problems to solve.

Becky shares some frustrations with her church.

The people who are active are very focused on what needs to be done. They are so used to solving problems that I think they tend to view people that way too. When people focus so much on my illness, I think that they fail to see me as a person. When people say, "What I want most for you is that you be healthy," I think that our relationship will always be strained. I am not healthy, and I don't know how to make myself be healthy. So when they insist that I should be, I feel like I'm failing in the relationship. What I want them to want most for me is that I feel loved and am able to reach out to others with God's love. I want to have peace and joy. If they could focus on finding ways to help me with that, we might be able to have a wonderful relationship.

Perhaps the most painful response from those who see the chronically ill as problems to solve is to detail things they assume the sufferers are doing wrong. A toxic illness sufferer with a perceptive father shares the following:

My dad says that people are uncomfortable when they see others suffering because they are afraid that maybe it means that suffering is a normal part of life, which would mean they might suffer too. So it's easy, when someone else is suffering, to try to look for something they are doing wrong or to offer solutions. Unfortunately, when this happens, the message that those of us who are going through hard times get is that we are not okay. Our experiences are not valid. We end up having to comfort and reassure people who we were hoping would offer us support.

After a while, the conversations seem less worth having. The following chemically ill people have reached that conclusion:

Corporate worship is very important to me. But lately the strain of dealing with the physical setting (chemicals) as well as the emotional setting (people who are so focused on healing that they can't help me deal with the reality I'm living in) has made it seem better not to go to church.

I recently met the mother of one of my daughter's friends. I was looking forward to meeting her as I don't know many people here in town. What I ended up getting was instructions on how I needed to be prayed over, have my house prayed over, get inner healing, and on and on. And of course how I really needed to come to church, despite my explaining why I could no longer go. I groaned. It's not that I don't believe that God can heal of course, but here was yet another person who was going to push me to do this and that, and very likely in the end would still insist that there must be something I wasn't doing right for me to still be ill. *Argh.* Been there, done that.

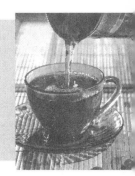

Take Care Tip

- Try to see people as people, and not as problems. Ask God to help you see the ill through his eyes.

BEATEN WITH THE BIBLE

Christians are as likely as the rest of the culture to believe on some level that people can will or think their way to health or that doctors can provide easy solutions. Christians, however, can add many layers to the message that people can avoid or easily address illness and that remaining sick is the sufferer's fault. These extra layers and the way they're communicated sometimes lead the ill to feel they're being beaten with the Bible.

Of course, many wonderful verses and stories in the Bible assure us God can and does heal. Most chronically ill Christians cling tightly to them and to the hope they offer. There are certain verses and statements, however, which others bring up so often when the topic of illness arises that sometimes people become defensive about them.

By his wounds we are healed. Isaiah 53:5 is often used to make the case that God has already provided physical healing for all and that those who are sick simply haven't claimed it. It speaks of the coming Messiah and states that by his stripes, or wounds, we are healed. There are various interpretations of this passage. Some, as noted, believe it means that physical healing is now available to all. Others believe it refers to the fact that Jesus would have a healing ministry on earth to validate his claim as the Messiah. Another view is that the healing referenced is the ultimate physical healing we will achieve when we shed our earthly bodies for glorified heavenly ones.

The interpretation many biblical scholars embrace and that makes the most sense to me is that the verse isn't referring to physical healing at all, but to spiritual restoration. Numerous verses in the Bible speak of healing in nonphysical terms such as the statement that God will heal the brokenhearted[182] or various proverbs such as Proverbs 15:4, which says that the tongue that brings healing is a tree of life, but a deceitful tongue crushes the spirit. Scholars point out that the context of Isaiah 53:5 seems to argue for this interpretation, as does 1 Peter 2:24, which says, "He personally carried our sins in his body on the cross so that we can be dead to sin and live for what is right. By his wounds you are healed."

Prosperity verses. Jeremiah 29:11 is another verse often quoted by those who believe in the universality of temporal, physical healing. It says, "'I know the plans I have for you,' declares the Lord, 'plans to prosper you and not to harm you, plans to give you hope and a future'" (NIV). Interestingly, in context this verse was a specific prophecy to God's people living in Babylon. God told them that they would be exiled for seventy years, but at the end of that time, he would bring them back to their land. There was hope in the message but no promise of immediate rescue.

The message, in fact, was just the opposite. Earlier in the chapter, in verse 5, God told the exiles to "plan to stay," and he specifically warned them against believing false prophets. From the context, it seems likely that the prophets were promising a quick end to the difficult situation. In verse 9, God said of those claiming to speak for him, "They are telling you lies in my name. I have not sent them."

In other words, the general message was something like this: "You're going to have to go through something you'd rather not, but don't despair. I'll be with you through it, and it will eventually end. Don't listen to the people who say you can cut the time short. This is part of my plan." It's ironic that, given this context, Jeremiah 29:11 is so commonly used to support the message that Christians should be immune from suffering.

There's another verse that uses the word "prosper" and speaks of health that is often quoted to those who are chronically ill. In the King James Version, 3 John 1:2 says, "Beloved, I wish above all things that thou mayest prosper and be in health, even as thy soul prospereth." To clarify this verse, let's look at it in context and in one of the many translations that make the message more understandable to modern ears. The NLT says, "This letter is from John, the elder. I am writing to Gaius, my dear friend, whom I love in the truth. Dear Friend, I hope all is well with you and you are as healthy in body as you are strong in spirit."[183] John was writing to a friend and saying essentially, "I hope you are doing well." It was a friendly greeting and fond hope but not a theology.

Did Jesus heal everyone? It's common to hear the statement that since Jesus healed every sick person he encountered during his ministry on earth, healing for everyone is a general principle that continues today. There are a number of responses to that statement. One is that of the moments in the life of Jesus recorded in the Bible, at least one indicates that he didn't heal every sick person he met.

John 5:3 tells us that there was a pool where "crowds of sick people" used to gather. People believed that the first person to enter the water after it was "stirred" would be healed. Jesus began a conversation with a man there who had been disabled for thirty-eight years, and the man complained that others always beat him into the water. It seems, from that statement, that the man was not for some reason alone at the pool that day. Evidently, people needing healing filled the area, but Jesus chose to heal only one.

Do physical diseases have spiritual roots? The Christian twist on the belief that those who are sick simply haven't claimed their wellness is that those who are ill don't have sufficient faith, don't know some spiritual principles, or have sin in their life that's blocking their healing or bringing God's judgment. (There seems to be a tendency among Christians to attribute our own struggles to spiritual warfare but to attribute the struggles of others to ignorance or divine discipline.) The story of the man by the pool seems to indicate that sin might have played a role in his condition. However, there's no indication that Jesus chose to heal him because he had cleaned up his life or had more faith than the others around him. Jesus told the man to stop sinning *after* he had healed him,[184] and the man evidently didn't have great faith in Jesus because he had no idea who he was.[185]

There's a pastor and author who has a ministry to people with various health conditions, including chemical illness, which is based on identifying and removing the spiritual roots of various diseases. Unfortunately, his approach has caused a divide in the Christian toxic illness community. Angela writes about her experience with his ministry.

> One of the hardest things is I had done the program years before he wrote a book. Then he wrote the book, and when it started to finally make the rounds in church circles, my phone started ringing. Well-meaning Christians on the other end of the line just "had" the answer for me for my healing. They were so persistent, and when I would tell them I personally met him and had done his program years ago already, they just wouldn't believe it; "'cause if I had, I would be healed!"
>
> Then the book became more popular, and my phone started ringing from acquaintances in my homeschooling group: more excited, well-meaning friends who were absolutely convinced that if I just did this and this and this, all would be well.
>
> You can't imagine how weary I became of having to give the news that I'd been there and done that. Their disappointment was more than I could bear, and I found myself having to manage their feelings on top of my own disappointed feelings, which were hard enough to bear alone and in silence, much less bear theirs, too.
>
> People mean well. It's hard for them to see us suffering, and they want to "fix" it. Often in their fervor to bring you what they perceive is relief, they can drive you nuts. It never seems to occur to any of them that perhaps you have been down every bumpy road, every trail that even offered

a glimpse of hope, turned over every rock, and are still sick. They are never convinced unless *they* were on the "journey" *when* you did it so they could *see* it for themselves. It seems my word was never convincing enough.

I guess that is what wore me out the most: each one wanting me to prove to their satisfaction that I had tried all the book had suggested. Only then would I be granted a reprieve from their incessant nagging.

But it's an ill wind that doesn't blow some good. Through this experience I learned to appreciate people who are aware. People who understand something when you tell it to them and they hear you. People who know that you know more about your own body than they do. People who appreciate you, and listen to you, and believe you when you tell them you've been there, done that.

I've had enough of well-meaning Christians who are undone by suffering and kick into hyper mode and bother you to death until they can "fix" you. I am not mad at them, but I do wish some would be more considerate and think past their own discomfort in our presence. It always felt to me that it was more about them needing to 'fix it' because they didn't know how to just sit and let it be, and be comfortable that some people suffer and some don't, and sometimes that is just the way it is.

Sometimes I just need someone who can sit on a swing with me and never say a word.

Blake points out a common feeling of those who've been urged by others to do the program and have done so, but haven't been healed.

It's so hard when you aren't healed after you have gone through a program like that. You feel like God doesn't care about you.

Another chemically ill person adds:

I did the program, too. Mostly I just don't talk about it or tell people unless they directly ask. I don't want to discourage other people who might find some help or hope there, but the bottom line is that it didn't bring me healing, and I don't want to have to explain that (how can I?), justify myself, or somehow prove my spiritual health. It's hard enough that one more thing failed. I just can't handle the condemnation of others because of it. Do they think I haven't asked myself over and over why God didn't use it to heal me? Do they think I haven't searched my soul as deeply as I can for any sin I can identify?

Is there a relationship between sin and suffering? I believe that the Bible teaches that there is, both in a general sense and sometimes in a personal and specific way. However, the Bible is clear that it isn't always the case.

The book of John tells us that the disciples of Jesus saw a man born blind and asked whose sin caused it. In John 9:3 Jesus answered clearly that "it was not because of his sins or his parents' sins." On another occasion, those around Jesus discussed the unpleasant fate of some Galileans, and Jesus asked, "Do you think those Galileans were worse sinners than all the other people from Galilee? . . . Is that why they suffered? Not at all!"[186] If toxic illness is a result of sin, perhaps it's the societal sin of putting profits and other considerations ahead of human health or of believing that man-made products are superior to what God has created.

Obviously, the message that personal sin is the cause of sickness is more prevalent in some faith traditions than others, but no Christian struggling with a chronic illness is immune from the accusation. If those who are ill don't get the message from their family, friends, or fellow church members, they'll surely get it from television, radio, or online sources. It permeates our culture and is often just below the surface, ready to bubble up.

Generally, a Christian who has been sick for months or years has turned over every stone imaginable in an attempt to regain health. This almost always includes large doses of prayer and spiritual soul-searching. Not surprisingly, the chronically ill often feel very wounded and frustrated by those who assume otherwise and who blame continuing illness on spiritual failure. The following chemical illness sufferers open their hearts to share their experiences:

> Right now I am tired of the emotional roller coaster being involved in my church seems to bring. So much so, I don't want to contact them to say I am really struggling. There are a few people claiming God is healing me. Interestingly, two of these people have significant health problems themselves. Mine are just more visible.

> The "God has healed you" lady from church came over and stood at my door until I let her in. She ordered me to stand tall. She said God said she was not to pussyfoot around because He's tired of that. I was in tears and felt completely overpowered. I believe I always stand tall in the Lord, whether I am sitting or lying in bed. For me standing in the Lord is about the depth of my faith, not how I stand physically. I am left confused. But God brought me through.

> I have been told by two women at church that God is going to heal me, and this has already begun. I have been feeling very down and not wanting anything to do with anyone from church as I spent most of the weekend in bed after the last confrontation. I've had enough. My spirit feels broken.

> I like being around people who believe that God is active in the world today and who actually expect to see him do great

things. I got tired, growing up, of people who tried to keep God in a box where His actions could always be predicted and were always "safe." But I think that people who expect that God will always act in dramatic ways have just put him in a new box. We need balance. We need to recognize that the world is complex, and God responds with complex solutions.

In Matthew 25, Jesus tells a story in which people are judged by how they treated their fellow human beings. He says that that ministering to or ignoring "the least of these" is comparable to doing the same thing to him. Verse 36 is enlightening. To those he rewards he doesn't say, "I was sick and you rebuked me for my lack of faith" or even "I was sick and you healed me." To those he calls righteous he simply says, "I was sick and you cared for me."

Take Care Tip

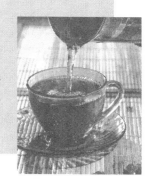

- Don't automatically accept other people's interpretations of Bible passages. (That includes any espoused in this book.) Study the Scripture for yourself and ask God for wisdom.

JUDGED LIKE JOB

A judgmental response to fellow human beings in pain isn't an isolated or new phenomenon and neither is the frustration and anger it can arouse. The Old Testament book of Job is a rich and beautiful observation of the nature of suffering. One of the many themes that unfolds is the relationship of those who suffer to those who observe and give advice. The story plays out as follows:

Job was a righteous and God-following man, but Satan accused him of worshipping God only because of the blessings God gave him. God gave Satan permission to test Job, within limits. He was allowed to harm him, but not physically.[187]

Satan attacked by killing Job's livestock, servants, and even his children. Job was filled with grief, but he fell to the ground to worship God and continued to praise him. Because Satan was unsuccessful in his attempt to persuade Job to abandon his faith, he asked God for permission to harm him further. He said in Job 2:4, "Reach out and take away his health, and he will surely curse you to your face." God gave his permission, and Job joined the ranks of the physically ill.

After Job lost his health, some of his friends came to visit. At first, they sat quietly and mourned with him. Eventually, though, they began to speak. Eliphaz was the first to make the connection between a righteous life and a lack of suffering. He seemed to suggest that if Job were truly righteous that God would quickly restore him. He suggested a prayer of appeal and urged him not to despise God's discipline. Job wasn't happy with Eliphaz's speech. He remarked that friends should be kind rather than accusatory, and he asked Eliphaz to stop assuming his guilt.

Bildad was the next to chime in. He echoed Eliphaz's assertion that if Job were pure and upright and would simply pray then God would come to his aid. Next, it was Zophar's turn. A different friend, but delivering the same message, turned up a notch. He said in Job 11:6, "Listen! God is doubtless punishing you far less than you deserve!" He counseled him to stop sinning.

Job's impatience and anger with his friends is clear in chapters 12 and 13. In Job 12:2 he says with sarcasm, "You people really know everything, don't you? And when you die, wisdom will die with you." He observed how easy it was for those at ease to mock those suffering and to "give a push to people who are stumbling."[188] He accused his friends of smearing him with lies, said that as physicians they were worthless quacks, and concluded that being silent would be the wisest thing they could do. The International Standard Version translates the first part of Job 13:5 this way: "I wish you'd all just shut up."

Job and his friends continued to trade barbs. Eliphaz tried to bolster his case by saying that others, older and presumably wiser, were on his side. He told Job, "There's no limit to your sins"[189] and accused him of a long list of specific ones. Job, for his part, told his friends they were horrible comforters and accused them of crushing him with their words, persecuting him, and chewing him up. In Job 27:12 he summed it up by stating, "You say all these useless things to me."

Modern-day toxic illness sufferers echo Job's response to his friends. Some examples:

> She starts down the faith healing and inner healing route . . . as if I haven't heard all this before, right? Bottom line is, I thought, "Here we go again!" It seems with all of that comes judgments and assumptions, doesn't it? After twenty-six years of illness, I've had my fill of trying to explain, feeling pressured and judged, etc. When I hear this stuff, I want to run for cover, *fast*!

> I was awakened by a phone call from one of the ladies from church who claims God has healed me. She said she will be visiting me in three hours on a mission from the heavenly father. I am not in the mood for false prophecy today.

> When we are sick, we are sick. We don't need anyone laying a guilt trip on us because we are not living up to their expectations. Ignorance is one thing. Cruelty is another.

> I don't let people get away with spiritual abuse anymore. Condemnation for my illness is not biblical in my point of view.

I get pretty upset when people tell me what God's will is for me. I'm confident that God can tell me himself.

———————

It sounds like people in your church are trying to force the world into a reality that makes them feel better, even if it's at the expense of your health and well-being. Maybe God wants you to help them mature spiritually, but I don't think he wants it to happen in a way that is damaging to you. Sometimes when people are being pushy, we have to push back.

The book of Job doesn't tell us how long Job suffered with his illness or with his friends, but the good news is that at some point God stepped in and met with him. He assured him of his presence and his sovereignty, and Job responded with humility and worship. God then turned his attention to Job's friends, expressing his own anger with their attitude and directing Job to pray for them. He promised to accept Job's prayer and not treat the friends as they deserved. After Job prayed for his friends, God gave him twice as much as he had before, then those who had known him previously came to his house and consoled and comforted him. The comfort and consolation were undoubtedly important aspects of the restoration.

Take Care Tip

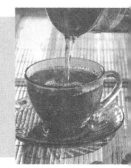

- Don't make spiritual judgments based on physical conditions. Beware of the tendency to associate suffering with the sin of the sufferer.

Pummeled with Prayer

Judgment of the chronically ill can manifest in many ways. Oddly and sadly, one of those ways is prayer. God acts through prayer and most people who are sick deeply desire the prayers of others. Unfortunately, however, there are occasionally times when prayer seems less like a weapon to use for fighting the forces of darkness and more like one to use for flogging those already weakened by illness. Many chronically ill Christians recognize that there's a difference between those who, out of love and mercy, pray for or with you, and those who pray *at* you. Kathy talks about the experience.

> Don't you just love it when people want to pray with you and then begin to ask God to show you all the sin in your life, increase your faith, deliver you from false beliefs so you can be healed, etc., etc.? Every word can feel like a knife.

It isn't wrong to pray for others to receive conviction of sins, become stronger in faith, or be delivered from false beliefs. However, when those prayers are prayed aloud and tied to the issue of healing, the message that sometimes comes through is one of condemnation rather than concern.

In Luke 18, Jesus told a story about two men who went to the temple to pray. One mentioned the other in his prayer. He basically said, "Thanks, God, that I'm not like that tax collector." The tax collector was mentioned in the prayer but not actually prayed for—the recitation was more about the one doing the praying. Sometimes prayers for healing can also seem more about the person praying than the one who has the need. Stacy shares her thoughts.

> I can't judge people's hearts, and maybe I'm wrong, but I get the feeling that sometimes people pray for me so that if I get well, they can get the credit for it. Generally, they're people who have just met me and then announce to the world that they are going to pray for me in a way that communicates that since they've come on the scene, everything is going to change now. Sometimes they tell stories about other people they prayed for who got well. I'm grateful for the prayer—I

truly am—and I'll leave judgments of motivations to God,
but there's something about the approach that disturbs me.

I believe that most of the time people pray with pure motives, true
concern, and active faith. Even in those situations, however, there are
possible pitfalls. One is that those who pray for you will sometimes express
disappointment or blame if they see no immediate answer. The following
chemically ill people had that experience:

> Ironically, prayer is what I want most from my Christian
> friends, but I also find myself really tensing up when some-
> one says they want to pray for me—especially in person. I
> can't count the number of times that people have prayed for
> me and then watched me like some sort of science project
> or asked me over and over again if I was feeling stronger.
> Yes, sometimes I've said I thought I was just because I knew
> that was the only answer that would make them happy. I
> just can't stand the constant feeling that I'm letting people
> down by remaining sick.

> I eventually became wary of asking people to pray for me
> because they can become so focused on the result rather
> than being supportive during the process.

> I want to make it clear I'm happy for people to pray for me,
> just not with me in regard to healing unless I specifically
> request it. Basically, I am happy for them to believe for my
> healing. I just don't want to hear about it anymore.

Another prayer pitfall is that sometimes "I'll pray for you" seems to include an unspoken "and don't expect me to do anything else." It's nice to be

prayed for when recovering from a chemical exposure, but it would certainly be better not to have been exposed in the first place. James 2:15–16 speaks about words and deeds that aren't in harmony. James says, "Suppose you see a brother or sister who has no food or clothing and you say, 'Good-bye and have a good day; stay warm and eat well'—but then you don't give that person any food or clothing. What good does that do?" A chemical illness paraphrase might ask, "Suppose you know a brother or sister has physical problems with your perfume or cleaning products and you say, 'I'm sorry you have that problem; I'll pray for you'—but then you don't make changes that could keep the person healthy. What good is that?" Julianne notes:

> I finally got up the nerve to talk to a lady at church about the problems I have with perfume. She said she would pray for me, but she didn't change her perfume use one iota. She obviously sees this as my problem and doesn't think it should affect her. It's kind of like running over someone with a car and yelling, "I'll pray for you" as you drive off.

Despite the occasional negative experiences, in general the chronically ill are extremely grateful for prayer. As mentioned previously, MCS sufferers found prayer among the three most helpful "treatments" rated.[190] When I think of the power of prayer, I often think of James and Peter, both disciples of Jesus and leaders in the early church. Acts 12 tells us that both were thrown in prison. James was killed, but Peter was supernaturally released. We aren't told why God chose to spare one and let the other die. The only clue is found in verse 5, which tells us that while Peter was in prison, the church prayed very earnestly for him. I don't believe the difference in outcomes was because James had sin in his life or didn't know some spiritual principles. Perhaps the difference was simply the prayer of God's people. Though prayers may occasionally cause discomfort, I believe that most people prefer any well-intentioned prayer over the option of not being prayed for at all.

Take Care Tips

- Pray for those who are ill, but avoid expressing condemnation or judgment in your prayers.

- Make prayer an addition to practical action, not a substitute for it.

- Try not to blame people who are sick if prayers for healing aren't immediately answered. Continue to pray. Chronic illness needs "chronic" (continuing) prayer.

DISAPPOINTED IN THE DIVINE

For a Christian, the hardest emotions to admit and express can be disappointment in and anger with God. I imagine all chronically ill Christians have experienced the types of feelings expressed below.

> Part of me is really upset that God hasn't chosen to heal me now and seems to be requiring me to go through a challenge that I would rather not endure. This goes back to a view of God that I got as a child when I was put in situations I wasn't prepared to handle and told it was God's will. When I'm in that type of situation now, I tend to think that God's up there nodding with satisfaction, saying, "This is exactly what I had in mind."

⎯⎯⎯ ⟡ ⎯⎯⎯

> I've realized that I have a sort of "antenna prayer" going up all the time—a sort of "Please God, please God, please

please please . . ." in the back of my head. I get upset talking about this, and I think that part of the reason is that it reminds me of areas where God has apparently not given me what I was asking for, at least not right away. I know all the "right" answers about why God sometimes doesn't seem to answer our prayers or doesn't answer them in the way we expect him to or think he should. But on an emotional level, I struggle.

Anger at God has a particular flavor that no other anger has. God is, after all, the one who truly, easily, and without a doubt could fix us. We may dare to be angry with him, but we don't want him angry with us.

There are many opinions about anger in general and anger at God in particular. I don't claim to have any special wisdom, but I observe a few things from Scripture.

Many of God's servants expressed their frustration and anger at God very openly. Our friend Job spoke as honestly and openly to God as he did to his accusing friends. He declared to God that he wouldn't keep silent, and he didn't. Among other things, he seemed to:

- blame God for his suffering (6:4, 7:20, 10:16, 13:24–25, 16:7–14. 19:21)
- believe that God had wronged him (19:6)
- wish God would leave him alone (7:19, 10:20)
- doubt that God would hear his pleas (17:7)
- express frustration that God didn't answer his cries (30:20)
- doubt that God would give him a hearing but expect to be crushed instead (9:16–17)
- feel terrified and afraid (9:34–35, 13:21, 23:15–16)
- wish he had never been born (10:18–19)
- have no hope (14:19, 17:15)
- be unable to rise above his pain (14:22)
- declare that his spirit was broken (17:1)
- believe God was unfair (21:7, 27:2)
- feel God was far from him (23:3, 8–9)

What did God think of Job's words? We have two messages to reconcile. One, found in chapter 40, verses 2 and 8, is that God seemed to rebuke Job for criticizing, discrediting, and condemning him. Job's response to his encounter with God was to say that he spoke of things he didn't understand, and to repent, although the Scripture doesn't explicitly tell us the nature of his repentance.

We find the second message in God's statement to Job's friends in Job 42:8, which was, "You have not spoken accurately about me as my servant Job has." Other translations say, "You have not spoken of me what is right" (NIV) or "You have not spoken the truth about me" (HCSB). What did God mean by that? Scholars have offered various interpretations. Some believe that God was saying that in the central matter of dispute between Job and his friends (the matter of whether or not Job was suffering because of his sin), Job's words were right and the friends' were not. Others say that Job's final words during his encounter with God were what God declared "right" or "accurate" (although he really said very little).

The explanation I find most intriguing is that the word translated "accurate" carries the connotation of "honest." In *The Message*, Eugene Peterson embraces this explanation and states verses 42:7–8 this way: "After God had finished addressing Job, he turned to Eliphaz the Temanite and said, 'I've had it with you and your two friends. I'm fed up! You haven't been honest either with me or about me—not the way my friend Job has.'"

Given this interpretation, it seems possible to me that the Lord's basic message to Job was something like "Job, you've said things about me that aren't true, and I won't leave the statements undefended, but I'm glad you've been honest about your feelings and kept the dialogue with me open." Job's friends, on the other hand, seemed to have talked more about God than to him.

As I've wondered through the years what is and isn't okay to say to my heavenly Father, one verse that has given me cause for caution is Philippians 2:14, which warns us against complaining. I was interested to learn that the original term used for complaining was *goggusmos*, which has been translated as "murmuring" and "grudging." One of its definitions is, "a secret displeasure not openly avowed."[191] Perhaps the message is that we need to guard against muttering under our breath against God or talking behind his back, so to speak.

Being honest with God forces us to be honest with ourselves. I believe that God wants us to drag our feelings into the light where he can address them and where we can look at them objectively. A real relationship, as opposed to a surface one, is almost certain to involve anger on occasion, but if anger causes parties to turn away from each other and close off conversation, the result can be devastating.

The Bible instructs us not to sin in our anger.[192] Anger can be the genesis for a long list of potential sins, including bitterness, hatred, rebellion, and revenge. Anger at God can lead to evil, but it can also lead to a deeper, more real and honest relationship with him. As one Bible study author notes, "God doesn't want our 'right answers'; He wants our hearts . . . even if they're a little explosive."[193]

Recently, an online friend stated that God tends not to answer our "Why?" questions. I believe he often does answer them, but as I began to reflect on what might cause him to be silent at times, I realized that often a "Why?" question is more rhetorical than real. Sometimes when I scream, "Why, God?" I don't really want information. I just want to be rescued. I think what I'm often really saying is something like, "I don't deserve this. You should treat me better." I'm like a two-year-old screaming at a parent, and God lets me rant but has no need to answer a question I didn't really ask. Sometimes "Why?" really means "Why?" and sometimes "Why?" actually means, "I'm mad at you, God."

The Bible doesn't hide the true emotions of believers going through difficult times, but an important lesson from Scripture is that men like Job, David, and other psalm writers who expressed their angry feelings freely didn't let anger completely define their experience with the Lord. In the midst of his other statements, Job said, "I know that my Redeemer lives."[194] The author of Psalm 10 began it by asking in verse 1, "O Lord, why do you stand so far away? Why do you hide when I am in trouble?" but ended it in verse 17 by saying, "Lord, you know the hopes of the helpless. Surely you will hear their cries and comfort them." Honesty began the conversation, and the open dialogue left room for God to respond and for the author to remember the nature of God's character. If we don't close the door on the relationship we have with our Father, we can find peace in the storm.

Take Care Tip

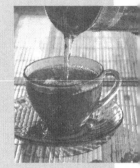

- Keep your relationship with God open and honest and pray that others will also not allow pain to close off true communication with him. Give yourself freedom to express your feelings, and allow others to do so, but allow God to speak as well.

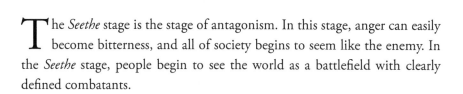

CHAPTER EIGHT

I am attacked by people I don't even know; they slander me constantly.
They mock me and call me names; they snarl at me.
—Psalm 35:15b–16

The *Seethe* stage is the stage of antagonism. In this stage, anger can easily become bitterness, and all of society begins to seem like the enemy. In the *Seethe* stage, people begin to see the world as a battlefield with clearly defined combatants.

INDIGNANT AT INDIFFERENCE

By the time people with toxic illness have reached the stage of antagonism, they've generally been sick long enough for those around them to tire of engaging with a problem that has no easy solution. As previously discussed, the problem-solving approach tends to involve steps such as suggesting doctors and treatments, praying, getting frustrated and angry that the challenge still exists, and "writing off" the problem by assuming that the ill have caused, made up, or exaggerated their situations. Another approach is to simply banish the problem from conscious thought, an approach that generally comes across as indifference.

The indifference of others to their plight is one of the things that can make those with toxic illness seethe. The simple truth is that people everywhere can make easy changes that would make a difference in their own lives and health and a huge difference in the lives of the chemically ill. The fact that they don't can be the impetus for much aggravation. People with toxic illness often believe that if anyone will make changes, their families will, but that isn't always the case as the following experiences illustrate:

> I can't go to my daughter's house since they use fabric softeners. If they would just change that, I could go there. They aren't willing. Who understands families? Only the Lord.

> I'm ready to scream. My family pressures me to attend family events but doesn't make much effort to make them safe for me. When I give in and go, I always get sick then they express frustration about that. It's like cutting someone and getting mad when they bleed.

The products that keep the chemically ill bound to their homes are so unnecessary that much resentment can come from that fact, as well. Carol says:

> I watch my husband go off to places we used to go together, and it's hard to believe I can't go with him just because someone will have perfume on or there are plug-in air fresheners there.

In the *Seethe* stage, there is a lot of irritation at society in general. The following comments seem to indicate that antagonistic thoughts often surface when watching TV:

> Why is it that after some people have battled MCS for twenty plus years, the harmful stuff is still being used in everyday products? Why aren't there lawsuits against these companies? Every time I watch a commercial on TV that promotes something that I am sure would be toxic I ask these questions.

I have been watching a TV program about the Australia zoo. They did a major remodel so that each animal has the environment that is perfect for them. I think I will sign up as an endangered species. They can put me in an environmentally safe cage. I will put on a show for people.

Some of the research into our illness is promising. I get mad, though, when I think about how long it has taken for it to get done. Then I see a commercial on TV for a new candy and think, "Just imagine if someone would put that same amount of energy and imagination into researching what's making me sick!" Clearly, resources are not being used very efficiently.

My children know if my TV screen is ever broken it's because I tossed something at an air freshener commercial.

The complacency of the church. Christians can have especially strong emotions at the seeming indifference of the church body. Some chemically ill Christians share their experiences.

I'm trying to figure out what to do about this group of ladies from church who have started meeting together. They invited me and said that they would come to my house, but then one lady called and said that they "couldn't" come to my house "for a number of reasons" and could I possibly come to her house. I have told her before that I have a problem with something in her house, but she insists that the only scented product she uses is "natural."

The fumes bothered me the whole time I was in her house. Eventually I started breathing through my jacket. At the end of the meeting one of the ladies said she hoped I would come again. I explained that something in the house was bothering me, and the lady whose house it was said again that the scented product was natural and she had taken it upstairs. Another lady said, "Would it help if we met at the church?" I said, "It would really help me if we met at my house." They didn't say that they would do that. If they could meet at the church, they could meet at my house. I wish I had had the nerve to say, "So what's the problem with meeting at my house?"

The use of so many chemicals, especially in church, is so upsetting for me. I feel banned.

In response to the request from my husband (the pastor) for a chemical free church, the most I get is, "I won't hug you because I have perfume on."

In the *Sigh* stage, the chemically ill try to make excuses for others. ("They don't understand. They just forgot.") In the *Scream* stage, sufferers conclude that very often the only explanation for people's actions is selfishness or indifference, and by the *Seethe* stage, they are sure of it. Sometimes it's almost impossible to make sense of people's behavior such as when doctors who claim to understand and treat those with chemical illness have offices full of synthetic fragrances and other toxins. It's also very difficult at times to understand the actions of church members and leaders. Rosie relates the following experience:

> The women's group at church invited me to come speak next month. They said they would go fragrance-free for that meeting. What this says to me is that they know their

products make me sick, they know why I can't come to the meetings normally, and they know they could make changes so I could attend. They are willing to make the changes so I can minister to them but not willing to make the changes so they can minister to me. Wow, that sure makes me feel loved.

The Aroma of Christ website related the following story shared by a reader:

I once asked my pastor to print a line in the bulletin requesting people use less perfume at Sunday services. I told him a friend of mine in another church had this done for her and it really helped. . . . But he said he "couldn't." Never knew why not. I set up my own "fragrance-free zone" in the cry room, leaving a $250 air filter in there set on low. If no one smelly was using the cry room for the service, I could attend but not receive communion unless someone who was "clean" brought it to me. I needed the filter left on, but the pastor kept turning it off because it "used electricity." I checked with the manufacturer, and they said it used about as much as a 25w bulb, pennies a month. He still turned it off.

Money is obviously not always the problem. I personally know of two situations in which people offered both funds and labor to construct a safe room, but church leaders declined the offers. I also know of other cases where people bought items such as conference phones or webcams to include the chemically ill in church activities, but the items were never used.

It seems possible to me that God might want to say the same thing to some church leaders that he said to some leaders of Israel in Ezekiel 34:2–6.

What sorrow awaits you shepherds who feed yourselves instead of your flocks. . . . You have not taken care of the weak. You have not tended the sick or bound up the injured. You have not gone looking for those who have wandered away and are lost. . . . So my sheep have been scattered without a shepherd, and they are easy prey for any wild animal. They have wandered through all the mountains and all the hills, across the face of the earth, yet no one has gone to search for them.

In the same chapter, in verse 18, God has words for some fellow "sheep." He asks them, "Isn't it enough for you to keep the best of the pastures for yourselves? Must you also trample down the rest? Isn't it enough for you to drink clear water for yourselves? Must you also muddy the rest with your feet?" When people are unable to attend corporate worship services because of toxic products others use, it can feel like the water of life has been muddied.

There are many ways that others may express indifference to chemical toxicity issues and cause much exasperation. Some examples:

I've actually had some people tell me that my problems were too big for them to hear about! Not help with, mind you, just to hear about. Somehow, hearing about them was more than they could handle!?? I was floored when I was told that.

My MCS is pretty severe, and it would take quite a bit for our church to be safe for me. I've come to accept that they aren't going to make those changes. What really makes me want to scream, though, is that they could make smaller changes (change cleaning products, for example) that would make a difference for a whole lot of people. Why don't they care about that?

The church says they want to attract people, but they put

up barriers that keep people out who desperately want to come in. It infuriates me. Who is going to reach these people? I don't think God is going to just look the other way. I can only imagine what Jesus thinks about the situation and what he would do if he were to walk in one of our toxic churches.

What would Jesus do? What does he think about barriers in the church? He showed us his thoughts and feelings on the subject when he drove the moneychangers out of the temple. They had set up shop in the Court of the Gentiles and were impeding worship for non-Jewish believers who had come to meet with God. Jesus made it clear that he wanted the house of worship accessible to all.

Take Care Tip

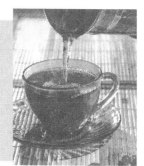

- Fight the human tendency to become indifferent to the plight of others. Ask God to make your heart soft.

FIGHTING GOLIATH

Chemical manufacturers. In the *Seethe* stage, the chemically ill have come to understand that the fight for recognition and help for toxic illness isn't just a fight against ignorance. Ephesians 6:12 tells us that our real struggle isn't against "flesh and blood," but against spiritual forces. On the physical plane, however, there is conflict with those who have vested interests in pushing the belief that MCS is an imaginary condition and that the products in our environment are safe. In an important and eye-opening article entitled "Multiple Chemical Sensitivities under Siege,"[195] Dr. Ann McCampbell states that since manufacturers are unwilling to acknowledge the message that their products cause harm, they attempt to silence the messengers instead and are behind a concerted campaign to cast doubt on the existence of MCS. Deception is again a weapon of choice. McCampbell states:

> To that end, they have launched a multipronged attack on MCS that consists of labeling sufferers as "neurotic" and "lazy," doctors who help them as "quacks," scientific studies which support MCS as "flawed," calls for more research as "unnecessary," laboratory tests that document physiologic damage in people with MCS as "unreliable," government assistance programs helping those with MCS as "abused," and anyone sympathetic to people with MCS as "cruel" for reinforcing patients' "beliefs" that they are sick.

Chemical manufacturers often take a page from the playbook of the tobacco industry by using nonprofit front groups with neutral, pleasant sounding names, third party spokespeople, and "science-for-hire studies" to try to prove that their products are safe and those who believe otherwise are delusional. The American Chemistry Council, then called the Chemical Manufacturers Association, launched their attempt to prevent the recognition of MCS in 1990. Their goal was to work through physicians and medical associations. The article notes that "the industry has enlisted the aid of vocal anti-MCS physicians who promote the myths that people with MCS are 'hypochondriacs,' 'hysterical,' 'neurotic,' suffer from some other psychiatric disorder, belong to a 'cult,' or just complain too much." These doctors work for the chemical industry as high-paid expert witnesses, but since they don't usually disclose their financial ties in their writings or speaking engagements, people are generally unaware that the opinions are not unbiased but reflect the chemical industry's agenda.

Interestingly, drug companies are also working to deny the existence of MCS. McCampbell explains that many companies that make medications also manufacture pesticides, which are widely implicated in causing and worsening chemical illness. The article names eight large and well-known companies that each have ties to both the pharmaceutical and pesticide industries.

Opposition from the pharmaceutical industry plays out in many ways.

One is that researchers supportive of chemical illness find it difficult to get their studies published in the medical literature. Because medical journals rely on drug advertisements for funding, they are hesitant to publish pro-MCS articles for fear of alienating their advertisers.

This dynamic affects other avenues of information sharing as well. Funding for the American Medical Association relies in large part on the sales of drug advertisements in its journals, and drug companies are major donors to the American Academy of Family Physicians. Doctors find it difficult to receive accurate information about toxic illness and are unprepared to deal with patients suffering from the condition. As a result, according to McCampbell, "their responses to MCS patients have tended to range from dismissive to blatantly hostile."

The pharmaceutical industry exerts its influence however it can. Despite being a major source of funding for medical research, they are not only failing to pursue research on chemical illness, but attempting to block research by others. The article notes that industry lobbyists commonly call for more research on MCS while simultaneously attempting to suppress it. They state that you can't prove it exists without more study, but that you can't study it because it doesn't exist.

McCampbell designates the Environmental Sensitivities Research Institute (ESRI) as the leading opponent of MCS. Its past activities include

- publishing newspaper advertisements made to look like legitimate news stories stating that MCS "exists only because a patient believes it does and because a doctor validates that belief"

- paying a medical journal to publish the proceedings of an anti-MCS conference that was partly organized by a firm owned by ESRI's executive director

- sending anti-MCS literature to a state disability agency developing a report on MCS, which included advice on how to avoid accommodating chemically sensitive employees

- sending a representative to a Medicaid Advisory Committee meeting to urge that Medicaid benefits be denied for the diagnosis and treatment of chemical sensitivities

- providing a representative to speak against MCS at a continuing medical education (CME) conference for physicians where he failed to disclose his industry affiliations as required by CME guidelines

- sending a member to speak to the staff at an independent living center where he berated them for providing a support group for people with MCS

The chemical industry is also very involved in suppressing the truth of chemical illness in the justice system through such avenues as filing briefs, supplying "expert" witnesses, and distributing anti-MCS literature to attorneys and witnesses. They've been influential in convincing many judges not to allow toxic illness testimony in court. This is despite the fact that, when McCampbell wrote her article, there were over six hundred articles on MCS and related conditions in the published literature, which, despite the chemical industry's efforts, supported a physiological rather than a psychological basis for MCS in a ratio of two to one. The scientific evidence is even stronger now, but the struggles for recognition continue.

The attacks come from every angle. In the last decade or so, the chemical industry has attempted to change the name of MCS to "idiopathic environmental intolerance" (IEI). The chemical lobby prefers the term because idiopathic means "arising from an unknown cause," so by adding that designation and removing the word "chemical" they can distance themselves from the condition. There are also escalating attempts to get medical licensing boards to revoke the licenses of physicians who diagnose and treat chemically reactive patients.

The chemical/pharmaceutical industry is powerful, well-funded, and relentless, and their attempts to discredit chemical illness and those who experience it have been largely successful. Those already suffering from a devastating illness continue to face hostility and scorn from those who should give them help. These facts should make any caring individual seethe.

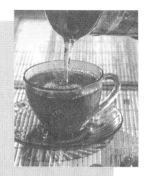

Take Care Tips

- When you read or hear something that denies the existence or seriousness of toxic illness, even if it comes from a seemingly respected source, be aware that vested interests may be behind the message. Don't accept everything you hear or read about MCS at face value.

- Be aware that when you buy toxic products, you put your money into the hands of those who are attempting to discredit the chemically ill.

Insurers. The chemical industry has greatly influenced another Goliath that the chemically reactive must face. The insurance industry (health insurance, worker's compensation, disability, etc.) has a large vested interest in suppressing the epidemic of chemical illness. Opposition from insurance companies has a huge impact on the daily lives of those reactive to chemicals because people with toxic illness are often in a truly desperate situation financially. In 2002, the Environmental Health Coalition of Western Massachusetts surveyed their members. They found that 10 percent had an annual household income of $5,400 or less, 35 percent made between $5,401 and $12,000, 22 percent earned between $12,001 and $24,000, and less than a third (31%) made over $24,000 as a household. Higher incomes correlated with living with a partner (presumably healthy and able to work). Seventy-five percent of those living alone had a gross income of $12,000 or less.[196]

Many toxic illness sufferers have trouble pinpointing when their condition began. Even those who had a significant precipitating exposure at work are often reluctant to claim worker's compensation. Ashford and Miller note that an attorney and executive editor of the *Ecological Illness Law Report* believes that only about 1 percent of severely affected chemically ill workers will file a worker's compensation claim because they don't want to be labeled as psychiatric cases. They also point out that many workers leave jobs because of chemical illness but are not able to tolerate their new jobs either and find themselves unable to file claims against either employer.[197]

The small percentage of the chemically ill that do take on the fight for insurance benefits often find themselves in a nightmare world. Teacher Lorraine Smith's saga is far too typical and is representative of thousands and thousands of others. Her challenges began with the first visit to the doctor the court ordered her to see.

Within minutes of entering the doctor's waiting room, which had no windows, Smith began to react to toxins, so for an hour and a half she managed her symptoms by repeatedly going outside and coming back in to see if the doctor was ready for her. When she was called back to a windowless examining room, she asked if there was an alternative room with a window and was told no.

After ten minutes in the examining room, Smith's breathing difficulties caused her to open the door to the hallway to get some air. The doctor passed by and shut the door, giving her an annoyed look. After a while, Smith opened the door again, and again the doctor passed by and shut the door. At that point Smith left the room and asked the receptionist how much longer it would be before seeing the doctor. The receptionist didn't know, so Smith went back outside to clear her system of toxins as much as possible. After another half an hour, the doctor was ready for her. Smith describes the rest of the visit.

> I went back into the stuffy little room. A man with intense eyes and wildly curly hair came into the room and shut the door. I didn't say anything because he seemed adamant about this door.
>
> [The doctor] smiled broadly. I wondered if he was very friendly. As the interview went on, I realized that he was laughing at me. When I described my symptoms, he chuckled. Other times he laughed. I finally mustered enough courage to ask him why he was laughing. He replied, "It's a long story." I asked him to tell it to me. He just shook his head and laughed. "No, it's too long." Then he

continued asking questions and he continued laughing at me. Although I tried to convey the seriousness of my illness and how desperately I was trying to survive, he just kept laughing.

Although Smith had called ahead to request that the doctor please not wear any fragrance, he was wearing aftershave lotion that caused Smith to feel weak and dizzy and have trouble breathing. When Smith mentioned her problems, the doctor laughed again and told her he was wearing a "special fragrance" that didn't cause sensitivities.[198]

Surviving mocking doctors is part of the fight. Another is surviving the courtroom. Smith's story continues with her description of appearing for her worker's compensation hearing.

> The courtroom was filled with people wearing fragrances. In order to receive my benefits, I had to be present. Nobody assisted me in any way. To avoid the fragrances, I waited for my turn in a small room, alone. Many hours passed.
>
> I realized then that, although the court pays lip service to environmental illness, it truly does not understand the condition. Part of the disability for a person with environmental illness involves great difficulty being able to be in public buildings. It is extremely hard if no provisions are made. In court, I needed the people present to refrain from wearing fragrances. It would have helped if I had had access to fresh air, perhaps an open window. Also, I should have been scheduled as the first case so that I could leave as soon as possible. Without these provisions, I was actually being asked to perform tasks that were the very nature of my disability. This has to change! Worker's compensation hearings should not involve an obstacle course so that if the person survives his court appearance, he might receive benefits. Certainly a person confined to a wheelchair would not be required to climb three flights of stairs to appear at a hearing! This would be utterly unfair. So, too, is it totally unreasonable to require a person who reacts severely to

the slightest of odors to endure a courtroom full of people wearing strong perfumes and aftershave lotions![199]

Smith was directed to return to "the laughing doctor." This time her husband accompanied her. She waited in the car and her husband came to get her when the doctor was ready. At this visit, she asked the doctor to please open the door to the examining room, and he asked her why. She writes:

> I tried to explain that I needed fresh air. He smirked and said that there was "air" all around me. . . . I was having great difficulty speaking, for my mind was affected by the lack of air. I remember telling him that I had no life and that I was suffering. He smiled again and said curtly, "You have a life. It's a life." This man amazed me. He was so cruel.[200]

As is usually the case, Smith's journey was full of twists and turns and ups and downs. At one point, she was awarded compensation but later ordered to pay it back. She was refused her pension because of a private meeting held with a doctor who had never met or examined her—a meeting neither Smith nor her attorney were invited to attend.[201] Smith speaks for all Davids who have battled Goliath.

> I broke down into tears again. . . . I just kept remarking that I could not believe how shabbily I was being treated. Why was I being deserted like this? I felt as if I were being left by the side of the road to die. Nobody cared! The only efforts being put forth were those meant to avoid any responsibility. For twenty years I had given so much of my energy to being the best teacher I could be. I had never asked for anything in my life before. The one time I needed help, everyone—the school, the doctor, the insurance company, and the court—just coldly turned their backs![202]

Take Care Tip

- Consider offering practical help to those attempting to qualify for disability or worker's compensation. Offer to write a letter of support, or help someone navigate a doctor or courtroom visit.

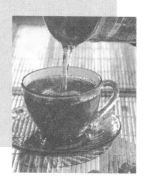

SCREAMING INTO THE WIND

The chemically ill often feel that one of their purposes in life is to play the role of canary and warn others of danger. Opportunities abound. Kelly shares about taking her car to have some work done and telling the workers how unhealthy the air in their shop was for them.

> They told me that my car wasn't finished yet because almost everyone in the garage had called in sick. They then mentioned that four guys in the shop had been diagnosed with mini-strokes and that one had actually died two years earlier. I offered to talk to their boss and bring in some information . . . . They both quickly said, "Oh, no, don't talk to our boss; we could lose our jobs."[203]

When efforts to inform don't seem to be working, it can raise strong feelings. These toxic illness sufferers express them.

> Everywhere I go, I meet people who are sick. It seems like there are more sick people than healthy ones these days. I try in every way I know how to warn people about the dangers of the products they use, but they refuse to take me

seriously. It makes me mad. How can you save people from themselves?

———••◆••———

My former employer is a bully. I am sad that nothing in that work environment has improved. I have a friend that is still there, and she's sick now.

———••◆••———

Have you seen some of the things that are being called "green" these days? Does it really make sense to save the earth but kill each other in the process? What's it going to take for people to get it? Question of the day: as a society, just how stupid are we? Answer: pretty stupid, evidently. Maybe we can blame that on the chemicals too. Our brains have all been so affected that sometimes I seriously wonder if it's almost too late to save ourselves.

Take Care Tip

- Listen to the message the chemically reactive "canaries" are trying desperately to communicate. Believe that toxic illness can affect anyone and beware of the natural tendency to think, "It won't happen to me."

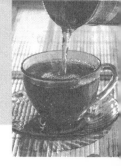

TAKING SIDES

The growing frustration with society in general and with seemingly uncaring people in particular can lead to the development of an "us versus them" mentality. Sharon talks about the phenomenon.

> There are many reasons and times in our lives when we find ourselves outside the group, but most of those times we have more choice in the matter. When it occurs because of symptoms from a health condition which we have no choice about, it is a totally different thing to deal with. From my observation, it is not "us" who separate from "them" or even initially see ourselves as different from "them," but it is "they" who see us as outside the group. After all, we "won't" conform to their ways, they think. Few ever think to adapt themselves to ours so that we can remain included.
>
> I've missed my baby's burial, my father's burial, my mother's funeral, my son's wedding, the birth of several grandkids, many school programs etc., etc. I wanted to go. I grieved not being able to attend. It's unbelievable to have someone telling you that you just don't want to go or something about not doing the right thing by not attending. After a while, you do feel like you are on the outside looking in. You're no longer one of "them."

Others illustrate the growing divide between "us" and "them."

> As for making new friends, I'm to the point where I just prefer meeting other Christians who also have MCS. It's just much easier to *not* have to try explaining and re-explaining all the time and still not be understood.

I am so tired of trying to explain this disease. And I am so tired of looks on others' faces that I must be nuts to believe that I even can react to fragrances. And I'm so tired of the attitude that if they don't tell me they are wearing a fragrance, I won't know and won't react. Sorry to be so down. My attitude hits bottom when I can't breathe. Right now, most everyone in my life feels like a difficult person. I have to keep reminding myself that God is still there, and he understands.

------- ◆ -------

There was an incident with my husband on Saturday. He wants to bring something that "might" be toxic into the house and "hide" it to see if I'll react when I don't know it's there. *Yikes!* What is he thinking? Sometimes I feel like a widow.

A particularly difficult circumstance is when the "them" in the equation live nearby as the following comments indicate:

I am sick from a neighbor who has been burning oil and rubber in an outdoor burner. I write him letters begging and even offer to pay him to burn clean, but the insensitivity of people like that is the hardest thing I have to deal with and that is the major cause of depression for me. They can call me oversensitive all they want, but they are cold hearted and under-sensitive to their neighbors. Loving neighbors is a Christian commitment, but they don't seem to think it applies to them. I pray every day for a cure for this horrible disease.

------- ◆ -------

My husband wants to move for fear of what our neighbor could do to me. I am getting hang-up phone calls now. I need prayers to help me. I am scared, and don't know what to do.

———•◦◦◦•———

Our neighbor is up to no good. I am afraid of him because I am alone so much. Anybody who can know he is making me suffer so much is capable of anything. Please pray that the Lord intervenes and stops him. Please pray hard for God to intervene.

Neighbor wars involving the chemically ill can involve suits and citations initiated by both the healthy and chemically reactive parties. Those who own their homes often feel unable to leave, but renters have left toxic situations and been sued for abandoning their lease.

Some with chemical illness ponder novel solutions for neighborhood issues.

I wonder if we could get the government to order pollution caps for dryer vents like they do the coal industry smoke stacks. Wouldn't that be great?

———•◦◦◦•———

If fabric softener fumes were green, then people would be able to see how far they really did travel. Pesticide fumes should be purple. Wouldn't that be quite the sight—purple and green air? At least, it might make people stop and think.

Those with toxic illness desperately want others to stop and think. The challenge of the *Seethe* stage is to remember that we're all being poisoned and all being deceived. Though it may sometimes seem like the world is divided into us versus them, we are really all in this together.

Take Care Tip

- Avoid the tendency to see the world in terms of "normal" people versus those with toxic illness. Remember that the fight is against deception, misinformation, and actual chemical dangers, not against each other.

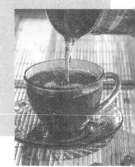

$\mathcal{S}$alvage

The Lord is my shepherd; I have all that I need.
—Psalm 23:1

After the antagonism of the *Seethe* stage, a person with toxic illness turns a corner. The next stage in the journey is the stage of salvaging health, meaning, and hope from the toxin-scarred life. God is in the salvage business, and he can restore the body, soul, and spirit.

BODY

The body becomes a constant focus of attention for the chronically ill, and like all who suffer physically, the chemically reactive desperately long for healing. Sometimes it occurs. Sometimes people regain a significant degree of healing and wellness.

As previously discussed, there's no single formula for fixing chemically damaged bodies since individual weaknesses call for individual repairs. One truth, however, seems clear: the earlier sufferers realize the chemical connection to their symptoms and begin to lighten the load on their detoxification systems by sifting and separating from toxins, the more likely their bodies are to heal and regain balance. To convey that message to those who are just beginning to experience chemical illness is an important goal for this book, and

I pray that those in that category take this message seriously. The canaries are chirping loudly. Please listen to their song.

Those whose bodies regain tolerance for everyday chemical exposures face an important question. How far should they push their detoxification systems? Unfortunately, toxins can cause internal damage that isn't readily apparent. Online toxic illness communities are full of stories of people who began reexposing themselves to substances they couldn't previously tolerate, only to later succumb to cancer or another serious disease. The "rain barrel" can be partially emptied, but it will always hold a finite amount.

Most people who regain chemical tolerance wisely apply hard-earned lessons and continue using nontoxic products and avoiding exposures as much as possible. Those who've made the toxic illness journey and come out on the other side also tend to be aware that they can send others down the same road by the products they choose to use. The bottom line is that there is never a good reason for *anybody* to use toxic products. Christians, who represent the body of Christ and understand their stewardship of this earth, should take very seriously the responsibility to do their homework and select products wisely. I believe that God cares a great deal about the products we use on the earth he created and the bodies he provided.

Take Care Tip

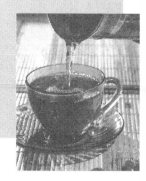

- Care for the body God has given you. Remember that chemical illness is much easier to prevent than to fix.

SOUL

Rebuilding support systems. Sometimes broken bodies don't get significantly stronger, but broken souls do. Often, this healing relates to restored and renewed relationships. This may involve family and friends who begin to understand needs, make changes, and advocate for the chemically ill. Some toxic illness sufferers share their stories.

I praise God I was able to attend my extended family Christmas party safely last night. Last year I had to leave in the middle of the party due to a reaction from someone's "secondhand" cologne on their shirt. It was so sweet—my mom thought of the idea of making a "fragrance-free room" for me in the event someone accidentally showed up with cologne residues on their clothes like last year. If that would've happened, my mom would've told the "smelly" folks to not come into the family room and that would've been designated as my "safe zone." Isn't that cool? I almost didn't come to the family party this year after last year's fiasco, but with my mom's support, I decided to risk it and things turned out great.

———◆———

Waiting for energy to return is so frustrating. When I am able to think it out clearly, I remind myself of how blessed I am to have a husband who values me for who I am rather than what I can do.

———◆———

Certain family members, who didn't understand what this illness really is, used to give me unsolicited advice that didn't help. I took that opportunity to try to explain to them what I was going through was more than "just allergies." Eventually they have become my greatest allies.

During the salvage phase, old support structures may be rebuilt. Others, though, may fall away while God raises new ones to take their place, as he did for these chemically ill people.

The hardest thing is not being able to make new friends since I'm not out in the world. A few months ago, I lost most of my physical support (and I only moved two miles), but God gave me three families willing to help in my new apartment. So I lost some and gained some. God does provide.

———⋅◆⋅———

I enjoy hearing about new modalities in medicine and new products as I've learned some useful, applicable, and practical things that way. But it's my decision as to whether or not I choose to embrace them or research it further. More often than not, I've already tried it and/or researched it for myself. I'd prefer to be informed about anything people want to share and then have them change the subject and move on to another topic. Yet, so many people start the unsolicited advice and kick into the fixing mode. I find people who have embraced some sort of suffering or obstacle in their own lives do not do this to me. They have a level of awareness that only suffering produces in one's life. They are a pleasure to know and make it worth all the effort to fellowship when I can.

———⋅◆⋅———

I remind myself that I do have reasons for hope. I am healthier now than I was a few years ago, and I have access to more and better medical care than I did when I first got sick. I have made moves, like joining email groups and starting a support group, that are designed to build a new kind of social network. But rebuilding does involve clearing the old structure away, and that in itself takes energy and resources.

Take Care Tip

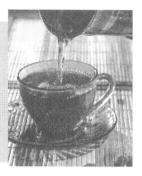

- Help be part of a rebuilt support system for someone whose old support structure has fallen away.

Accepting limits. Clearing the old structure away is important in salvaging the soul. In practical terms, this involves accepting limits. When to release specific hopes and dreams for the future is a very personal choice, for hope is a great source of strength. Holding onto desires that seem less and less achievable, however, can also sap strength. Many people find relief in letting go of specific goals so they can focus on other, more realistic ones. The following chemical illness sufferers have found freedom in changing expectations:

> I've been dumping files of teaching stuff, no longer hoping to get back into it somehow. What a relief to accept reality, clear out the impossible, and get on with the future.

> In the fall, I signed us up for ballroom dancing lessons. What was I thinking!!??!! I lasted two sessions and that was too much. It only made me feel worse, physically and emotionally. Physically because the perfumes overcame me and the activity was too demanding. Emotionally because I still saw myself as eventually becoming the person-in-retirement that I had always envisioned. Lately we have realized that we need to develop new hobbies (that aren't so active or

social), and individual interests rather than expecting to do everything as a couple.

People who say to "get on with your life" are blind to what your life is. Accepting your limitations *is* getting on with your life. Bemoaning your fate and trying to do the things that are socially acceptable but unachievable would be getting "stuck" in life as far as I see it. "Stuck" in the past if you will. Unable to let go of what you've lost. I'm sorry that others don't understand.

There was a time I was struggling to stay in a Christian grad school, which was newly built and had a poor ventilation system. My health was deteriorating, and I was trying to keep up with my studies, but I kept getting symptoms. A friend asked me on the phone, "Why do you keep doing this?" It jolted me. I quit grad college, and my life has taken a huge turnaround—mostly in the area of creativity. I finally gave up trying to make things happen, which were not suitable for me at the time. It's always hard and a loss when I need to quit before one of my goals is finished. I'm grateful, though, that I made the choice to leave the academic life, at that point. My blessings have been abundant in the midst of, and probably even because of, this horrible illness.

It's natural to think of hope for the future and acceptance of current limitations as opposites, but not seeing the two as incompatible can provide a significant degree of peace. Many who've struggled with trials have realized that it's possible (albeit challenging) to both accept what life has to offer today, and, at the same time to hope, pray, and work toward changes for tomorrow.

God's instruction to Israel in Jeremiah 29 illustrates the concept. As previously noted, he promised the exiles living in Babylon that he would bring them back to Jerusalem after a set amount of time. He assured them he had plans to give them a future filled with hope. He didn't give them false assurances, however, that the exile period would quickly end. Instead, he told them to make lives for themselves in Babylon. He instructed them to build houses and settle down, plant gardens, marry, and increase in number. In other words, he told them to believe in and count on a changed future but to accept current reality and make the best of their present situation. I believe he instructs us all to do the same.

Take Care Tip

- Pray that the chronically ill will know which goals to retain and which to let go.

Discovering gratitude. For the chronically ill, accepting current reality can be hard for many reasons. A significant challenge is missing former activities and relationships. Some have salvaged that truth by realizing that people only grieve for things that were meaningful to them, and the fact that we grieve is proof that we've had full and joyful experiences. Ashton says:

> I've been making a conscious effort these days to turn thoughts of what I can no longer do into prayers of thanks that I was able to do those things once. Thanking God for that, and for the good that still exists in the middle of this crazy life, has really made a big difference in my mental well-being.

Most of us want to know God's will for us, and in some matters, he makes it very clear. First Thessalonians 5:18a says, "Be thankful in all circumstances, for this is God's will for you." Philippians 4:6 tells us that thanksgiving is to accompany our requests to him.

Why does God want us to be thankful? Well, for one thing, it's good for us. Gregg Easterbook reports that "people who describe themselves as feeling grateful to others and either to God or to creation in general tend to have higher vitality and more optimism, suffer less stress, and experience fewer episodes of clinical depression than the population as a whole." He notes that "these results hold even when researchers factor out such things as age, health and income, equalizing for the fact that the young, the well-to-do, or the hale and hearty might have 'more to be grateful for.'"[204] Giving thanks doesn't mean denying pain. It simply means acknowledging that pain isn't all there is and that God and his provisions for us are bigger than our trials.

One way that some toxic illness sufferers have found to embrace gratitude is to view their lives from a global perspective, as these people do.

> I remember clearly several months ago being in my cozy little "car bed" just considering and pondering. At first, I began feeling sorry for myself. Then, I remembered my husband telling me that when he went to Africa several years ago, the people at a tribe he visited had only one blanket and a wooden thing they used for a pillow. No house, not even a hut! As I lay there under my cozy 100 percent cotton blankets, warmed by the ceramic heater in the back seat, looking at the beautiful stars through my car's windows, feeling ever so secure in my little locked car in my friend's driveway, I realized how many blessings I should be thankful for! I wasn't cold, wet, unsafe, afraid. No snakes would crawl over me, no bears would attack me, no one could get into the car with all the doors locked. Even though it was a bit unconventional, my "ironing board" bedframe worked like a dream! Most of all, I knew God had His hand upon my life and was my protector and provider.

I have a greatly restricted diet, but I often remind myself that I probably still eat more in quantity and variety than an enormous amount of people in the world do. (I also think about the Israelites who ate manna day after day.)

Take Care Tip

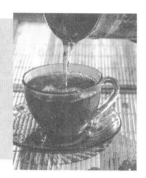

- Embrace the power of gratitude. Model it in your life and let others find strength in your example.

Extracting purpose from pain. Salvaging a life affected by chronic illness not only means accepting current limits and learning to be grateful for aspects of both the present and the past, but also involves the essential task of finding purpose in pain. To find purpose in suffering is to go beyond making peace with circumstances to embracing the truth that pain can be the genesis for positives not likely to be birthed from a struggle-free life. Whatever else it may include, for the chemically ill, this generally involves realizing that toxic illness has led to acquiring knowledge about common products and their negative effects that most people haven't felt the need to acquire. Most chemically ill people conclude that they must share this knowledge. In the *Salvage* stage, antagonism turns to activism. Avery states:

> I don't know how many times I have said, "Lord, you have my attention. What do you want me to do?" God says that I have a big mouth and will tell everyone about MCS.

Fortunately, in some cases, people are listening to the canaries chirp. The next chapter will deal with progress.

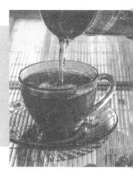

Take Care Tip

- Pray that none of us will waste our pain but will find purpose in and through it.

SPIRIT

The body and soul can be salvaged, and so can the spirit. The responses of God's people to those broken by illness can greatly aid or inhibit their spiritual restoration. To represent God on this earth is a serious and solemn trust. However, no matter what God's people do or don't do, true spiritual healing and growth can never come without time spent in communion with God. It's challenging, in our busy society, to carve out the necessary space away from people and activity to focus on God and spend time with him. In that area, the chronically ill may have an advantage as the following toxic illness sufferer has learned:

> Life can begin all over again with new ways to celebrate, new relationships, new things to appreciate, and, best of all, time to spend with the Lord, just you and Him. I spend much more time sitting and working in the yard just enjoying nature in a way I've always loved but didn't have time for before. God be with all of us as we change our lifestyle, keep close to him, and appreciate what we can still do.

Lane agrees.

> I believe that through my illness, God wants to teach me total trust in Him—that is, without any humans in between him and me.

Ridings recalls that the apostle John was banished to an island where God revealed to him the writings we now know as the book of Revelation. In that spirit, she keeps a note posted to a table at the end of her bed that says, "MCS is my island of Patmos where God can speak to me."[205]

People are fallible, but God is not. In Ezekiel, God condemned both shepherds and fellow sheep for mistreating and abandoning weaker members of the flock. God promised, however, not to leave them to fend for themselves. In Ezekiel 34:15–16 he says this: "I myself will tend my sheep and give them a place to lie down in peace . . . I will search for my lost ones who strayed away, and I will bring them safely home again. I will bandage the injured and strengthen the weak."

Although those confined to their homes because of illness may have an advantage of a sort when it comes to spending time alone with God, most quickly learn that discipline is still required. It's easy to fill the days with other activities, thinking there will always be time later for Bible study and prayer. Communion with God doesn't automatically accompany solitude. I once read, however, that in order to hear the "still, small voice" of God the listener must be even stiller and smaller. The homebound and chronically ill may have a head start on those attributes.

God works with us individually and personally, but there are lessons undoubtedly common to most of his children who suffer from toxic illness and other chronic conditions. Some of the common lessons are these:

Unanswered prayer doesn't mean God isn't listening or doesn't love us. One of the most important spiritual lessons for the chronically ill is that unanswered prayer doesn't mean God has abandoned or stopped loving us. I'm using "unanswered prayer" in the manner commonly used—for prayers that don't receive an immediate "yes" response. However, we have to admit that "no" and "wait a while" are indeed answers—just not the ones we want.

For a clear example of the fact that a "no" answer isn't related to God's love for us, we need only look to Jesus in the Garden of Gethsemane. Approaching the hour of his arrest, he asked (perhaps pleaded with) his father to change the plan, praying in Matthew 26:39, "If there is any way, get me out of this" (MSG).[206] God said no. He didn't change the plan, but he allowed Jesus to experience excruciating pain, passing through the horror and shame of beating and crucifixion. Had God abandoned, forgotten, or stopped loving his son? Of course not. The temporal suffering was for an eternal purpose. Love meant paying the price of sacrifice for an outcome worth the cost. It was *because* of God's great love that he didn't bypass the suffering of Calvary.

The fact that God loves us is generally one of the first spiritual lessons most of us learn—at least on a cognitive level. "Jesus loves me," we sing. "This I know." Indeed, we do think we know that truth, but to truly internalize it, especially during times of unanswered prayer and prolonged suffering, is something that the Bible says goes beyond our human knowledge and takes God's power. Ephesians 3:18 says, "May you have the power to understand, as all God's people should, how wide, how long, how high, and how deep his love is." We need power to really understand it. We simply can't fully comprehend it on our own.

At this point, we come to a paradox of continued suffering. When we first enter a time of pain and unanswered prayer, the natural response is to feel abandoned and unloved by God. As we continue to walk through the valley, however, we become more and more aware of the paucity and inadequacy of our own human resources. We realize we are dust. Slowly we learn to draw on God's power rather than our own limited supply, and, wonderfully, when we substitute God's power for our own, we find not only strength to face the storms, but the power mentioned in Ephesians—the power to truly understand and fully experience God's love for us. God's power gives us the strength to stand firm in suffering. It also gives us the ability to understand his nature. We need God's resources to truly grasp his love for us, and we most trust in and appropriate those resources when we come to the end of our own.

There's another reason God's love can become more real to us during prolonged pain. In such times we often become aware of the limitations to the human variety of the emotion. We understand that others seem just as selfish as we are and that they often seem to love and value us conditionally—for what we can do for them or for how we can enrich their lives. Sometimes recognizing the limitations of human love causes us to reach out for the unconditional love that can only come from God. Cameron writes:

Over and over again, people say that their churches didn't want to make changes "just for me." Why not? Why aren't we important enough to them? There's no answer. The good news, though, is that Jesus values me enough that if I were the one lost sheep he talks about in the Bible, he would have come looking "just for me."

Truly, there are truths about God's love we can't learn during times of ease. Only in times of suffering can we learn that God's love for us is wider, longer, higher, and deeper than all of our pain and distress and that he can strengthen, comfort, bless us, and answer many of our prayers while, for his own sovereign reasons and purposes, deny or delay answering some of the deepest cries of our hearts. It's a hard lesson to learn but once learned is a truth on which we can build and around which life can begin to make sense. God has not abandoned us any more than he abandoned Jesus on the cross, and his love for us is as deep and real as his love for his "only begotten Son," even when his perfect will doesn't include immediately answering prayers for relief and healing. When we suffer, we reach out to God—and find him, in the words of the poet Alfred Tennyson, closer than our breathing and nearer than hands and feet.[207]

The fruit of the Spirit can grow in all kinds of weather. The fact that the creator of the universe truly loves us is foundational, and when we embrace that knowledge, our desire to please God and become more like him increases. Every day all believers have opportunities to develop spiritual muscles, water and tend the fruit of the Spirit, and grow in likeness to our Savior. Just as physical muscles develop with resistance, so too pressure and pain may enhance our spiritual growth. Misunderstood chronic conditions like toxic illness may provide us with a rich spiritual training ground as Hayden points out.

> A family member shook his head at me and said he was sorry I was treating myself the way I was in avoiding things. It takes grace to not reply to such things, and perhaps we need to be grateful in some way that we are learning to practice the fruit of the Spirit in these times.

As we strive to become more like Christ, perhaps nothing is more important than learning to forgive as Jesus did. In the early stages of toxic illness, sufferers tend to think that those who cause harm by the products they use are simply uninformed. Gradually they become seen as selfish and uncaring, and by the *Seethe* stage they have often become the enemy. The *Salvage* stage is the one in which sufferers accept that selfishness is a universal trait, that God paid an enormous price to cover us with forgiveness and that he fully expects us to extend that forgiveness to each other. We continue to educate and advocate for change, but we view others as fellow sinners, covered by God's grace just as we are, and we forgive them.

The great hope in the story of Job, who suffered so deeply, is that God returned to him more than he had lost. It's important not to miss a detail, however. Job 42:10 says, "When Job prayed for his friends, the Lord restored his fortunes." His friends, of course, had wrongly accused Job of suffering because of hidden sin and had showed an enormous lack of sensitivity and compassion. God wasn't pleased with them, and he told them so, but he also said that he wouldn't treat them as they deserved but would accept the prayer of Job on their behalf. Why involve Job in the restoration of his friends? Perhaps because prayer for his friends was also part of the restoration of Job. He had to let go of the cruel things his friends had said to him. He had to let God judge their actions and not claim a right to judge them himself. He had to forgive, as do all who find themselves in similar positions.

God is really all we need. Forgiving isn't easy to do in our own strength, but 2 Peter 1:3 tells us that "God has given us everything we need for living a godly life." We've been given all the power we require to live godly lives, and, equally importantly, we've been given all we need for life itself. Philippians 4:19 tells us simply that God will meet all our needs.

This bold claim should lead us to consider a very important question. What, when we boil away all the nonessentials, *do* we need for life? We have physical, emotional, and spiritual longings. What are "needs" and what are not?

Physically, we need food, water, oxygen, and protection from disease and injury to keep our bodies alive. Emotionally, we feel a need for things like love, companionship, and peace. Our spiritual needs include a relationship with our creator and a sense of belonging and purpose in this world.

In truth, all needs are contained in one. When the biblical Martha complained that her sister Mary was listening to Jesus teach instead of helping with dinner preparations, Jesus told her in Luke 10:42, "There is only one thing worth being concerned about. Mary has discovered it." What we truly need is a relationship with our creator. A relationship with God meets our deepest spiritual needs and provides a means for him to meet our other needs as well. God made us—body, soul, and spirit—and he knows how we function. He owns the cattle on a thousand hills[208] and can easily provide for us.

Jesus speaks to this issue in Matthew 6. He reminds his audience that God feeds the birds and clothes the flowers and that we are worth far more to him than birds or flowers. He states in verses 31–33, "Don't worry about these things, saying, 'What will we eat? What will we drink? What will we wear?' These things dominate the thoughts of unbelievers, but your heavenly Father already knows all your needs. Seek the Kingdom of God above all else, and live righteously, and he will give you everything you need."

Physical "needs" are hard to define because the effects of sin have touched the current bodies we live in, as they have the rest of creation, and they won't last forever. Fragile bodies are part of the effects of the fall of man. At some point, our bodies will fail, but this is necessary because, as 1 Corinthians 15:53 tells us, "Our dying bodies must be transformed into bodies that will never die." In a very real sense, our most basic physical need is to eventually trade in these temporal bodies for new ones. Sometimes God provides for our bodies now, while we're living on the earth, but sometimes he provides by gathering us to himself where a new body awaits.

God promises to meet *all* our needs. This includes emotional needs as well. Not only does God give us love, but He *is* love.[209] How about companionship? He promises never to leave us or forsake us.[210] He also promises to give us rest[211] and a peace beyond what we can imagine or understand.[212]

A spiritual lesson common to those with chronic illness is that the great "I Am" is enough. When the Israelites wandered in the wilderness, God provided them with manna, which was able to sustain them completely. If they had been regularly consuming meat, vegetables, fruits, and grains along with the manna, it's doubtful that they would have really believed that manna itself was sufficient to meet their needs. In the same way, we're tempted to use temporal crutches to try to prop up our souls and spirits. Only when they fall away do we discover there is an eternal source of strength that can hold us up without any other aid. Adrian notes:

> I never believed I was relying on anyone but God until God began to remove from me the things in which I was putting my trust. Friends fell away, then family members, then my job, then worldly success, then financial security. After each falling, I had to reevaluate my priorities and look deep into my heart. I realized I *had* been placing my trust in worldly things. I'm grateful to God for revealing my heart to me, for forgiving me, and for truly being my all in all.

In 2 Corinthians 12:7–9, Paul writes the following:

> I was given the gift of a handicap to keep me in constant touch with my limitations. Satan's angel did his best to get me down; what he in fact did was push me to my knees. No danger then of walking around high and mighty! At first I didn't think of it as a gift, and begged God to remove it. Three times I did that, and then he told me, "My grace is enough; it's all you need" (MSG).

God can use us, even in our present condition. God's power and grace are sufficient to sustain us and sufficient to take what we offer in weakness and turn it into strength. Another common lesson learned by those who face chronic illness is that God can use us whenever we are willing to let him and in whatever physical condition we find ourselves.

After I became ill, I began to read familiar Scriptures with different eyes. At one point, I was reading about Jesus and the woman of Sychar (the woman at the well) and several things struck me that I hadn't pondered previously. The story, related in John 4, says that Jesus was tired from the journey, so he sat down to rest while his disciples went into town to get food. Why did he rest while the others ran the errand? Was it simply that devoted followers wanted to serve their master, or was Jesus more tired than the rest of them at that point? The story continues by saying that after the disciples returned with food they urged Jesus to eat. Why were they so concerned that he eat?

Could they possibly have been worried about him because he seemed a bit "under the weather?"

The Bible certainly doesn't explicitly make that point, and I don't want to read more into the Scripture than is there. The Bible does clearly say, however, that Jesus was tired from the journey. The fact is that his physical state was less than optimal at that time, but it didn't keep him from having a significant and lasting ministry in the area.

Our physical limitations certainly don't limit God's power as the story of Samson illustrates. He destroyed Israel's enemies only after he became blind.[213] Paul, who ministered despite his own handicap, compared our bodies to jars used to contain God's light. In 2 Corinthians 4:7–10, he penned these beautiful words:

> We now have this light shining in our hearts, but we our-
> selves are like fragile clay jars containing this great treasure.
> This makes it clear that our great power is from God, not
> from ourselves. We are pressed on every side by troubles,
> but we are not crushed. We are perplexed, but not driven to
> despair. We are hunted down, but never abandoned by God.
> We get knocked down, but we are not destroyed. Through
> suffering, our bodies continue to share in the death of Jesus
> so that the life of Jesus may also be seen in our bodies.

The less able we are to minister in our own power, the more obvious it is that God's power is at work in us, and the more likely it is that God will get the glory he deserves.

Toxic illness sufferer Christina Sollenberger wrote of how the condition shattered her ministry goals when she became housebound, but she pointed out that the prophet Ezekiel was also housebound for a period of time. She noted that God directed Ezekiel to shut himself inside his house for a while[214] and pointed out that the strategy was "not exactly your Evangelism 101 ap-proach to missions." Sollenberger went on to say that "if our illness remains, God's purpose for our lives stands."[215]

Cindy Duehring is perhaps the most well-known example in the chem-ical illness community of someone whose life and work touched the world despite her severe reactions to chemicals. Growing up, Cindy was healthy, happy, and accomplished. She filled her life with music, church activities, and sports. She was valedictorian of her high school class and planned to be a doctor, so she began premed studies at a Lutheran university.

In her final year of study, Cindy's life changed forever when fleas infested her apartment, and she called an exterminator for help. The exterminator assured her that his bug bomb was so safe "a baby could lick it off the floor."[216] That statement was obviously a bit of hyperbole. After the pesticide application, Cindy began to experience problems like fever, nausea, diarrhea, and seizures. Eventually she was diagnosed with pesticide poisoning and was forced to abandon her studies and return to her parents' home.

Although her health continued to deteriorate, Cindy was able to be out in the world enough during those years to meet and marry her husband Jim. Their brief church wedding included an oxygen tank draped in silk flowers. After the marriage, Jim and Cindy moved into their specially built, low-toxicity home, with ceramic tile floors, stainless steel counters, and metal, glass, and hardwood furniture. Every room was equipped with a high efficiency air filter.

Although the home was a sanctuary for Cindy, it wasn't enough to keep her from deteriorating. She became more and more ill and reactive to the world as she dealt with unavoidable exposures and the damage already done to her central nervous system and internal organs. To the symptoms already experienced, she added extreme pain and kidney and respiratory effects, including anaphylactic shock.

Eventually, Cindy could no longer leave her home because breathing unpurified air triggered a bronchial shutdown. Jim served first as a minister, and later as a teacher at a Christian school. Eventually Cindy's health reached the point that Jim had to spend the week in a small cabin in order to protect his wife from perfume and detergent residue picked up from being out in the world, and he was only able to see his wife on the weekends.

It wasn't Cindy's suffering or isolation that makes her story unique, but how much she turned them into, like Rumpelstiltskin turning straw into gold. She founded EARN, the Environmental Access Research Network, which was considered the world's leading support advocacy organization for the chemically injured. Duehring answered about five hundred information requests a month, researching specific questions on medical and legal issues from doctors, scientists, and the chemically ill in thirty-two countries. She wrote a monthly profile of studies for one newsletter and published a bi-monthly compendium of medical and legal briefs for another. At one point, a government body commissioned her and the director of the Chemical Injury Information Network to write a white paper called "The Human Consequences of the Chemical Problem."

Cindy's limitations increased over the years, and eventually she was doing all this while unable to use a computer, fax machine, typewriter, or even telephone. In fact, any sound at all caused seizures, so she lived her life in silence. She relied on the help of volunteers with whom she communicat-ed by writing directions in longhand. Faxes and mail were delivered to her husband's cabin.

In 1997, Cindy received Sweden's Right Livelihood Award, commonly known as the alternative Nobel Prize. She received the award for "putting her personal tragedy at the service of humanity."[217] Jim flew to Stockholm to accept the award on her behalf. At that point, Cindy had not left her home at all for eight years.

Cindy Duehring's faith was what sustained her. She spent much time praying and reading the Bible. She said she often thought of the words Martin Luther's wife reportedly uttered as she was dying: "I shall cling to Christ like a burr."[218] Cindy died at the age of thirty-six, two years after receiving the Right Livelihood Award. Undoubtedly, her true reward was falling into the arms of her Savior and hearing, "Well done, my good and faithful servant."

Cindy Duehring's accomplishments are inspiring, but they can also provoke feelings of inadequacy in those who feel they can't contribute to the world the way she did. The truth is that God can use anything at all we give him in faith and trust. One toxic illness sufferer shares that perspective.

> When days get long, I get bored and feel useless. I remem-ber the paraplegic at the pool of Bethesda who could only lie on his mat waiting for the waters to be stirred where he thought he might be healed. Jesus used him to show His power over sin and death by healing him. To this day, people everywhere who read that story are inspired to trust

Jesus to take care of them too. I can sure do more than lay around waiting to be healed, but even if that's all I could do, Jesus can use that too.

Several years ago, I made a trip west to see my sister. Many years had already passed since I had been able to enter a church building for worship, but she informed me that her church had a rarely-used "cry room" with a glass front and a window that opened to the outside that she thought might make it possible for me to attend the worship service. I donned my mask and gave it a try.

I remember many things from that service, which was an oasis in my continuing journey through the desert of separation from the body of Christ. My most enduring memory, though, is of singing the song, "Potter's Hands" and being struck by the line asking God to "set me apart." I was in a separate room from the rest of the congregation, tangentially part of the service, yet not quite among them. I already felt quite "set apart" and wasn't sure I wanted to ask God for more of that.

As I pondered those thoughts, God spoke gently to my spirit, and I heard these words: "Remember that set apart doesn't mean set aside." Set apart doesn't mean set aside—a simple truth, but profoundly meaningful to me at that time. What does it mean to be set apart? It means to be separated for a different use—chosen for a different purpose than what is most common. As I continued to sing, Darlene Zschech's beautiful lyrics took on a new depth of meaning: "I know for sure all of my days are held in your hands, crafted into your perfect plan." Yes, I still believed that. "Teach me dear Lord to live all of my life through your eyes." Yes, I wanted and still desire to see myself as God sees me—as separated for a purpose, crafted by the Potter's hand, and set apart for his own use. Set apart but never set aside.

This world is not our home. A final lesson commonly embraced by those with chronic illnesses is that this world is not our true home, but just a temporary stop on the way to our eternal future. Suffering gives us a hunger for heaven, which helps us to live focused on eternity.

Philippians 3:20–21a encapsulates our hope. The apostle Paul says, "There's far more to life for us. We're citizens of high heaven! We're waiting the arrival of the Savior, the Master, Jesus Christ, who will transform our earthly bodies into glorious bodies like his own. He'll make us beautiful and whole" (MSG).

Our weakened, imperfect bodies will be made glorious and beautiful and, as Revelation 21:4 points out, when God makes his home among his people, there will be no more sorrow or crying or pain. For those living comfortable lives on earth, heaven may seem far away—something to ponder more seriously later as age advances. For those who struggle here, the promise of heaven can become a hope that surrounds and sustains, providing perspective on life and strength to get through difficult days.

The perspective gained by a focus on eternity can manifest in various ways. It can mean learning to care more about pleasing God than about pleasing the people around us, and putting time and treasure into things with eternal value rather than into things that will fade away. When we focus on eternity, the struggles of this life, real as they are, recede in importance.

The focus on eternity was what enabled Paul, who was beaten, stoned, shipwrecked, and arrested, and who evidently lived with a chronic physical limitation, to state in 2 Corinthians 4:17, "our present troubles are small and won't last very long. Yet they produce for us a glory that vastly outweighs them and will last forever!"

Christians may differ a bit on specific matters of theology, but this is what I believe is the core of the Christian faith. God created human beings to have fellowship with him, but when the first humans disobeyed their creator, sin broke their perfect relationship[219] and ushered in pain, death, and the promise of judgment.[220] We've all inherited a sinful nature and are sinners ourselves,[221] and because God is holy and sin isn't compatible with his holiness, sin must be addressed for the relationship to be restored.[222]

Our only chance for a restored relationship with God is for someone to pay the price of our sin for us. Since only a perfect person, who didn't owe a debt for his own sin, could pay the price for the rest of humankind, God sent his son Jesus to earth to live as a man and take our punishment as his own.[223] Jesus lived a sinless life, died in our place, and rose from the dead, conquering death for us all. Because Jesus lives, we too can live forever in the presence of God.[224] God highly values our free will and won't force us to have a relationship with him. We must make the choice to believe and trust.[225]

Faith in Christ involves realizing that we need salvation, understanding we're incapable of saving ourselves, and turning from trust in our own goodness to trust in the sacrifice of God's son. We can ask for and accept forgiveness from God and get to know him by reading his word and conversing with him in prayer as he helps us grow in holiness and gives us the peace and strength we need to navigate this imperfect world.

During these years of isolation, I've developed a new love for the description of God given in Genesis by a woman who undoubtedly felt very alone, abandoned, and mistreated. She had an encounter with God, which Genesis 16:13 describes like this: "Thereafter, Hagar used another name to refer to the Lord, who had spoken to her. She said, 'You are the God who sees me.'" Those of us with toxic illness and other chronic conditions may often feel invisible to the world, but God sees us. God's people will always fail to reflect God perfectly, but I pray that they will come to see us too.

Take Care Tip

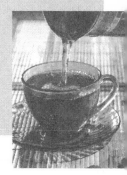

- Pray that those who are ill will have a deep and meaningful relationship with God that is continually growing and is a source of strength and comfort. Pray that they will understand God's immense love for them.

CHAPTER TEN

Smile

Fix your thoughts on what is true, and honorable,
and right, and pure, and lovely, and admirable.
Think about things that are excellent and worthy of praise.
—Philippians 4:8

The final stage of the chemical illness journey involves realizing that much about our society is dangerous and frustrating for those who understand the toxicity of common chemicals, but there are also signs of hope and progress. In the *Smile* stage, people see the positives as well as the negatives. It's the stage of taking encouragement from forward movement.

AWARENESS ACTIVITIES

Conscious change begins with awareness of problems and understanding courses of action that could alleviate them. To that end, activists have designated May as MCS Awareness Month. Of course, raising awareness should be an ongoing process, but human nature being what it is, it's often helpful to have a designated time to focus our energies and attention on a given matter.

Awareness Month activities are varied and diverse, but setting up educational displays is a common way to meet the goal of sharing information. During one awareness month, twenty-eight Ohio libraries provided information and displayed books related to the topic. They made a copy of the policy on indoor air quality from the Center for Disease Control available and urged people to adopt it. The US government has issued a number of helpful publications, including a guide for building owners and managers that covers maintenance, cleaners, "air freshener" products, personal care products, pest control, and more (such as the issue of vehicles idling near air intakes).[226]

People wishing to raise awareness have often found public libraries helpful in educating visitors about chemical toxicity issues, but educational displays can be set up almost anywhere. Health food stores and malls are good locations. How about a church lobby or a church library? Ridings provided a display at a pastors' conference.

Toxin-related health conditions are not just an American problem. Chemical illness is a global epidemic, and raising awareness of the issue should be a global undertaking. As part of awareness month activities in Spain, toxic illness sufferers submitted photographs of themselves wearing masks to a photo contest, and a popular TV show discussed the issue.

Those who wish to set up displays or otherwise focus more intensively on educational efforts during awareness month don't have to "reinvent the wheel." There are materials available to share, both secular and Christian. See the resource section for materials that can be printed or purchased.

Take Care Tip

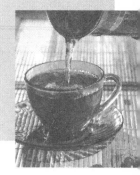

- Do your part to raise awareness of chemical illness and toxicity issues and consider using awareness month as a springboard or motivation. Encourage the efforts of others who are trying to make a difference.

FREEDOM FROM FRAGRANCE

The issue of synthetic fragrances seems one that more people, organizations, and even cities are taking seriously. An article in Connecticut's *Hartford Courant* notes that Halifax, in the Canadian province of Nova Scotia, was one of the first cities to engage in a "war on perfume." A university athletic center banned perfumes as far back as 1991, the hospitals are fragrance-free,[227] and at least two area churches have addressed the issue. The author notes that "when St. Michael's Catholic Church reserved a perfume section . . . and a non-perfume section, people from other parishes switched to St. Michael's."[228]

Another city ahead of the curve on the issue is Shutesbury, Massachusetts, which has long considered fragrance-free public meetings an important aspect of accessibility.[229] Actions include fragranced and non-fragranced seating at their annual town meeting and fragrance-free hours at the public library.[230] Even Las Vegas, not a city traditionally known for moderation or restraint, proclaimed a fragrance-free day in which leaders asked people not to wear perfume and hoped that they would use vinegar instead of some cleaning supplies.[231]

In her informative book, *The Case against Fragrance*, Kate Grenville writes that an employee in Detroit won a lawsuit against her employer for not providing her a safe work environment and that "within a week, the City of Detroit brought in a fragrance-free policy in all its workplaces."[232] She notes that the Centers for Disease Control and Prevention has made all its workplaces fragrance-free, as has the US Census Bureau and "many other organisations, big and small, public and private." She reports that when asked if they would support a fragrance-free policy in their workplace, 2.7 times more people reported they would vote yes than those who would vote no.

Of course, information and even policies are empty without corresponding action, but encouraging signs exist that consumers are beginning to vote "no" to fragrances with their pocketbooks. A *New York Times* article entitled "The Sweet Smell of . . . Nothing" notes that consumption of fragrances is declining. The author quotes beauty analyst Karen Grant. She states that "people are shying away from fragrances not for the traditional reasons that you'd expect . . . . Many people said it bothers them that fragrance has an effect on other people, that they are trying to be considerate by not overcoming others with scent."[233] Unfortunately, fragrance trends seem to be a good news/bad news situation. Home fragrances, such as sprays, plug-ins, and scented candles and oils, continue to increase in popularity.[234]

Take Care Tip

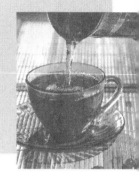

- Believe that when you go fragrance-free, you're on the leading edge of positive change. Set an example and trust that others will follow as people become more aware of the issue.

SAFER SCHOOLS

To safeguard and preserve the health of future generations, it's vital to address the issue of school air quality. Fortunately, some schools are doing just that. A study for the *Journal of School Health* found that 51.4 percent of schools had a formal indoor air quality management program.[235] Policies and programs undoubtedly vary widely in scope and true effectiveness, but looking at the issue is a vital step. A number of schools have instituted fragrance-free policies, and the American Lung Association offers a sample policy for schools wishing to adopt one.[236] Problems with enforcement have been noted at fragrance-free schools, but having an erratically enforced policy may be a step ahead of having no policy at all.

Cleaning products and practices are another area in which certain schools are beginning to make healthier choices. At Westmoreland Elementary School in Kansas, the staff noticed that all of the commercial cleaning products they were using displayed a label warning "Keep Out of Reach of Children." Wisely, they also noticed that most so-called green cleaning products they researched had the same label. They continued to search until they found a cleaning product in which all ingredients were on the Food and Drug Administration's "Generally Recognized as Safe" (GRAS) list.[237]

Pesticide usage in schools is an extremely important issue that more and more schools are beginning to take seriously. The "Best Control" nontoxic pest management program reports that their safe, alternative pest control program is already in effect in over 350 schools. An employee at a school in Michigan tells of treating a yellow jacket infestation in a ceiling unit ventilator with a combination of cardboard, a wet vac, water, and a little dish soap. He noted, "The result was all the yellow jackets were dead in the bottom of the vac. Before . . . we would have sprayed poison into that unit vent, ultimately exposing everyone in that room to some really bad stuff when the unit was turned on. We would have been putting kids in harm's way without even realizing it."[238]

Some schools are looking at toxins outside their buildings as well as inside. The governor of New York signed a bill banning the use of pesticides on school playing fields and daycare playgrounds. The bill has limitations (such as allowing chemical treatments to combat pests like rats and mosquitoes and only banning pesticides on playing fields and playgrounds, not surrounding green areas), but any step to reduce the toxic load is a positive one. Every step forward proves that change is possible with persistence and continued education. More than 18,000 people signed petitions in favor of the bill, which had previously failed to escape the state Senate nine times. A reporter noted that pest management companies, pesticide manufacturers, and landscaping and lawn care groups had donated tens of thousands of dollars to lawmakers over the previous years.[239]

Perhaps more school districts will make the switch to nonchemical yard treatments after looking at costs. A reporter noted that during the first two years of making the change, New York schools might see a slight increase in costs, but that annual costs should fall between 7 and 25 percent after the third year. A group called Grassroots Environmental Education offered free training to school groundskeepers on ways to care for fields without pesticides.[240]

In the past, the seriously chemically reactive have had very few options for schooling. A school in Washington provided such an option for more than a decade.[241] It began in the home of a teacher whose daughter was chemically ill, designed to be a safe haven for her and other students. Although the school closed its doors after eleven years partly due to the sale of the building they leased, the fact that they attracted enough students to operate, despite high tuition, demonstrates the reality of the need. Perhaps their example will inspire others.

Take Care Tip

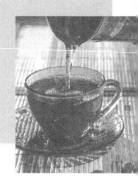

- Be encouraged by the efforts of governments, school boards, teachers, and parents to make schools healthier places to learn. Be part of a wave of change by advocating for healthy practices in your local school district.

HEALTHIER HEALTHCARE

Healthcare facilities are another place where changes in the toxicity of products used are greatly needed. Fortunately, a few organizations are taking the issue seriously. Health Care Without Harm is a global coalition working to reduce pollution in the health care sector. Their website contains information and fact sheets on cleaning products, pest control, and fragrances, among other topics.[242]

The Massachusetts Nurses Organization has been ahead of the curve on the issue of synthetic fragrances in the healthcare setting. In 2006 they published an article in their newsletter which discusses fragrance chemicals and their health effects, provides a model and sample of a fragrance-free policy, and includes a section on how to advocate for a fragrance-free policy in a healthcare environment. Elements of the proposed model include training for all staff on the adverse health effects of fragrance, along with distribution of a pamphlet suggesting acceptable personal care, laundry, and cleaning products. Patients and visitors are also to receive a pamphlet explaining the policy and how to comply with it. The model suggests that facilities place signs at entrances saying, "Welcome. This is a Fragrance-Free Health Care

Environment. For the health and comfort of all who use this facility, kindly avoid using fragrance."[243]

One hospital that aims to be fragrance-free is Women's College Hospital in Toronto. Their website states that they displayed posters near every elevator and in many clinics "promoting some of the things most important to our patients and their families—equity, privacy, patient affairs, and the WCH fragrance-free policy." They developed a poster displaying various perfumes and personal care products labeled with names like "nausea," "headache" and "wheezing," which informed that "fragrances don't smell beautiful to everyone" and asking people to respect the hospital's fragrance-free guidelines.[244]

Some hospitals in Maryland are trying to reduce the toxic load of patients another way—by addressing their pesticide usage. The *Baltimore Sun* reported that health care and retirement centers, including Johns Hopkins Hospital and the University of Maryland Medical Center, are working to eliminate toxic pesticides from their pest control efforts. Environmental advocates say it is the first effort of its type in the country.[245]

Take Care Tip

- Give positive feedback to any healthcare facilities or practitioners that are addressing the issue of air quality and chemical safety. Let them know the issue is important to you.

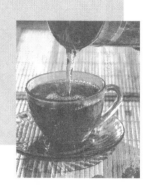

PROGRESS WITH PESTICIDES

The overuse of pesticides is a global problem, and some locations are taking it more seriously than others. In Canada, various municipalities began regulating the use of cosmetic (lawn) pesticides, and by the end of 2010, the entire provinces of Quebec and Ontario had restrictions on their use.[246] Lawn care in the United States is getting healthier in some locations. A

Seattle Post-Intelligencer article reports on using goats for weed control in the city of Auburn and notes that "from New England to the Southwest, goats and sometimes sheep are nibbling across areas heretofore dominated by the chemical industry."[247]

The road that leads to a nontoxic future is very long, but maybe we're at least facing the right direction. An *LA Times* article pointed out that natural and nontoxic products are no longer seen as part of a fringe lifestyle but are now mainstream. It quoted Morris Shriftman, former vice-president of a company developing less-toxic products, as saying, "We accepted this stuff blindly for so long. Now we're asking questions, seeking information. The awareness that we're living in a chemical environment is finally taking hold."[248]

Take Care Tip

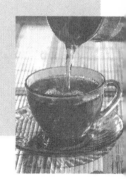

- Advocate for healthier pest-control practices and encourage those who have the same goals and are working toward them.

CHURCH CHANGES

The issue of church accessibility is such a huge source of pain for chemically ill Christians that they tend to greatly appreciate even small steps in the right direction. Some people share their victories.

> I actually got my church to use a nontoxic cleaner on the carpets recently. It worked great!

Before we moved, we were part of a small group that a lady who had MCS already attended. I didn't realize how much groundwork she had already done or how unusual it was to find a group of people who were so committed to doing what it took to allow us to participate. I am sure that group had a lot to do with my making it through those early months.

———◆———

My church finally has the webcast working on a semi-consistent basis. I can't tell you how much more a part of the church I feel when I can watch the services as they occur. It's not like being there, of course, but it's a huge improvement over the complete isolation of the past few years. I may still be invisible to them, but at least they're no longer invisible to me.

———◆———

My pastor put Romans 14:13 ("Make up your mind not to put any stumbling block or obstacle in your brother's way") in the weekly church bulletin to try and get people to refrain from wearing cologne and perfume to services.

———◆———

I know of churches where the bulletin asks people not to wear perfume. Of course, people are still going to be fragranced with other things, so it might not be enough for those of us who are pretty sensitive, but it's great for people who aren't as sick as we are yet. I really appreciate the churches that least take that first step and I really believe God will bless them for it.

———◆———

Just when I get discouraged about the lack of accommodation in churches, the Lord seems to give me some positive experiences again to keep me going! Last Sunday was amazing. When a couple who wore cologne a few weeks ago tried to sit at our table at Bible study, a man who knows of my perfume sensitivities spoke up and said to the couple, "Sorry, this is a fragrance-free table!" I couldn't believe it. I was so blessed that this man stood up for me! The couple said, "Hey, no problem. We didn't wear cologne this week." About a month ago, this same couple came and sat at our table, and I had to change tables immediately as the lady was covered in cologne. I guess after I moved, the other folks at the table explained why I left, so it looks like this woman doesn't wear perfume to church now. PTL! I'm so blessed by what appears to be her sensitivity to the issue.

This illness is a real roller coaster where sometimes we get so much love and compassion and other times it seems people don't care about our needs. I guess we have to tie a bow on the moments and memories when people go out of their way to accommodate us! Let's pray we all get more accommodation times like these! :)

Some churches, denominations, and Christian organizations have begun trying to educate their members about toxic illness and the chemical problem. The Anabaptist Disabilities Network devotes a section of their website to MCS,[249] and in a resource about accessibility issues, the United Methodist Church included information on access for the chemically sensitive.[250] The Christian Council on Persons with Disabilities also includes a section on Environmental Friendliness in their publication, "How Accessible is Your Church?"[251]

Safe rooms. Although the numbers are still small, a handful of churches are reaching out to the chemically ill in tangible, significant, and effective ways. Provision of a chemical "safe room" is one such way. A safe room can take various forms, but at its heart it's a room that keeps toxins out but allows participation in worship. Generally, it's a room at the back of the sanctuary, with a glass wall or large window facing forward, which ideally has its own entrance and ventilation system. Some churches have modified "cry rooms" designed for mothers of small children for the purpose. Some positive experiences:

> I went to church this morning and my pastor had made up some signs to post on the doors of the room they have set aside for us. In big red letters at the top, the signs said: "Warning." Then below that in black they said (also in big letters): "Fragrance-Free Zone." Below that in smaller print it said something to the effect of, "This room reserved for the chemically sensitive."

> My pastor has such a good heart! I am so thankful for his willingness to go to bat for the chemically ill. I was surprised that my church has worked so quickly to get this room up and ready for us to use—my head is spinning as this has all happened so fast.

> Wednesday night my husband went to Bible study and the associate pastor was praying. He said something like: "Lord, as I saw the people behind the glass on Sunday, I was remembering the lepers in the Bible who were cast aside by society as unclean. Then I realized, we are really the unclean ones."
>
> Wow! Is that too cool? The Lord is already showing people the truth here. All of a sudden, I got a vision that perhaps someday we will all be out in the main congregations of churches and the fragranced people will be behind glass. How do you like that picture? It reminds me so much

of the smoking issue. Smokers have slowly lost their rights over the years, and let's continue to pray that the same thing will happen with fragrance wearers—that the folks who don't want to be around it will start outnumbering the folks that do. Then we can all have safer, cleaner air to breathe.

Evidently, at least one church took that approach. In an article on the limitations of fragrance-free rooms, Don Hooser mentions hearing of a church with a "fragrance" room for those wearing perfume.[252] That forward-thinking congregation has undoubtedly learned that when churches make changes to accommodate the "canaries," it positively affects the health of all church attendees. In fact, many toxic illness sufferers who've convinced their churches to lighten the chemical load have noticed positive changes in the congregation. Jim wrote:

> A friend said she managed to get most people at her church to stop wearing fragrances and noticed after the change that there were very few people seeming sleepy during the sermons like there used to be. The connection is obvious to us, but they probably just think the sermons are getting better.

Fragrance-free services. While some churches segregate the perfumed from the non-perfumed within the same worship service, others have started providing for specific fragrance-free services. The AP reported on a Catholic parish in Minnesota that provided incense-free Christmas mass following requests from parishioners.[253] The good news is that the church provided the mass. The bad news, and a sign of how much our society needs to learn about this issue, is that one news outlet put the story in their "strange news" section.

Specific fragrance-free services are a great step forward. Other compassionate and loving churches have gone farther and do their best to make *every* service safe for those who react to synthetic fragrances. In an article in the *Anglican Journal,* entitled "Scent-free Parishes in Vogue," a church leader points out that "Liturgy is supposed to be life-giving, not life-threatening" and states, "I have problems with people deliberately choosing to make worship space unfriendly and life-threatening to people with [health] problems."

He points out that lowering barriers to worship for some disabilities, such as for those in wheelchairs, involves a capital cost, but that going scent-free costs nothing. The same article mentions another church where there are signs at the entrance and notifications on the website and in the bulletin stating that the church "strives to be a scent-free church so that services and events may be enjoyed comfortably by everyone." The church leadership reported no resistance to the congregation taking that step.[254]

In an article headlined "Chemically Sensitive Find Sanctuary in Fragrance-Free Churches," Joseph Heimlich, of Ohio State University's School of Environment and Natural Resources, speaks about the importance of churches taking action. He states, "Churches are often a place where people are paying attention to things they may not pay attention to elsewhere. If something comes to them from the pulpit, or the altar—from that authority—they'll hear it in a way they won't hear it from newspaper, radio, TV, or from someone else." He adds, "Also, in a religious community, you are caring about the other people in that community. Cleaning your environment, cleans it for everyone else too."[255]

Ministry beyond the church walls. Churches that see the chemically ill through the compassionate eyes of Jesus will try to minister to people in the areas of their greatest needs. The Barrhaven United Church in Ontario, Canada, tackled one of the greatest needs of toxic illness sufferers when it helped create a corporation that built a housing project that included seven safe homes for people with chemical illness.

The church worked hard to make the project a success. Phillip Sharp, the project architect, took an active role in making sure the units were built safely. He reported that it was surprisingly easy to get manufacturers to modify their products for necessary changes. The church worked with the neighbors, informing them of the needs of the chemically ill, and with the city and regional governments who agreed not to use chemicals on the surrounding lands, roads, or nearby baseball field. The city even agreed to cut the grass near the houses with a hand mower.

Sharp said he realized that the location of the units wasn't ideal for a toxic illness housing project, but he thought it was important to provide something for people unable to move to the country and build their own safe homes. He listened well to the message the canaries tried to communicate.

An article in *Peace and Environment News* reported that he now feels "morally obliged" to design healthy buildings because he realizes that any one of us could become hypersensitive. He stated, "I'm really concerned that we do it for everybody."[256]

Another example of the church ministering outside its walls involved a chemical illness sufferer in Michigan with housing needs. The city of Jackson took him to court because he failed to paint his home in compliance with a city ordinance. He faced the usual toxic illness hurdles of finding a safer paint and affording to have the work done, since he was unable to do it himself. The possible penalty was up to $500 in fines or ninety days in jail. Fortunately, a safer, low-VOC paint resolved the dispute, applied by the World Changers, a group of Christian youth volunteers. The homeowner called the ministry a "very big blessing" and said, "I have hope again."[257]

We need to make buildings, including homes, schools, hospitals, stores, and churches, less toxic. However, if the weather is cooperative and the outside air is good, a toxin-free church doesn't need a building at all. Linda Reinhardt became chemically ill from a mosquito pesticide aerially sprayed outside an open window in the room where she slept. She eventually recovered a large degree of health and completed a seminary degree. Afterwards, she and her husband moved to a remote area where she began a ministry to the chemically ill that she named the Jeremiah Project.[258]

The name for Reinhardt's ministry came from the fact that the prophet Jeremiah wept when he warned people of danger and they ignored his message. Reinhardt noted, "As part of my ministry, I warn people about the health risks of synthetics. People are dying from them, and I feel anguish in my soul when they don't listen." The project included a tape ministry, support groups, newsletter, and educational materials. It also included worship services—held outdoors. An article in *Presbyterians Today* described it this way:

> At the open-air services of the Jeremiah Project at Canyon Lake, worshipers sit under a grove of scrub oaks on park benches. Their view encompasses woods, canyons, and a rough cross made of cedar. Their pastor stands on a flat rock to preach.[259]

Unfortunately, two years after starting the Jeremiah Project, Reinhardt became extremely ill when a neighbor installed two tanks of diesel fuel on his property. It eventually forced her to flee her home. Previously she had estimated that about 30 percent of the people involved with the ministry were homeless or displaced from their home of choice. She joined their ranks, living in an isolated campground with no electricity or running water.

Linda Reinhardt passed away during the writing of this book. Specifically, she died at the very hour that I was meeting (outside) with my friend Debra, who was giving me her input on this chapter. Debra had read about Linda and remarked that it was a shame that her ministry was on hold. We discussed the fact that those with toxic illness have the knowledge and will to take on those sorts of ministry efforts, but they don't have the health and energy. We talked about the vital need for well-informed, healthy advocates.

The day after our conversation, I learned that Linda had died at the very time my friend and I were discussing her, and I wondered if there was a message in the timing. I believe there is. Perhaps the message is simply that the task of educating people about the danger of common chemicals, and of ministering to the chemically ill, is too big for any one person, but is achievable if we all do our part and work together. When I heard of Linda's death, I suddenly saw the task as a relay race, and I felt as if someone had just handed me a baton. If you've read this far, maybe you've been handed a baton as well. The analogy is imperfect because in this race many runners can, and should, run at once. Will you join the effort? The race is important. In many respects, it is truly a race for survival.

During the years she held her outdoor services, Reinhardt made a point of reminding those in attendance of others unable to be present. She followed a Jewish custom of filling a bowl with salt water to represent the tears of the absent. The basis of the custom is Psalm 56:8, where the writer says to God, "You have kept record of my days of wandering. You have stored my tears in your bottle and counted each of them" (CEV). Many of God's people continue to wander. How long must that continue? How many tears must continue to fall?

Take Care Tips

- Be on the front lines of change and take the lead in making your church healthier for all. Educate others and enlist their help. If you've read this book, you're already more knowledgeable about the chemical problem than most people in church or society today, and God can use you to make an enormous difference in the lives of many people. Be a good steward of the knowledge you possess and actively seek to expand your knowledge of the issue.

- Every church and public building should do the basics such as switch to fragrance-free nontoxic cleaning supplies, remove "air fresheners," and renovate and repair with nontoxic products. There's no good reason to dirty the air inside a church building, and I don't believe it pleases God. Nontoxic alternatives are available.

- Many churches should do much more such as provide a "safe room" for the severely chemically ill to use or provide a separate worship time for them. I believe there should be at least one Christian church in every geographical area that is possible for toxic illness sufferers to attend. People with chemical illness are often desperately hungry for spiritual and emotional support and how you treat them and meet or ignore their needs may influence their lives and future immeasurably. If attending a Christian church isn't an option for the chemically ill, where will they go and how will they fill the spiritual void instead? Jesus tells us in Matthew 25 that ministering to others (the "least of these") is like ministering to him and that, conversely, failing to minister to them is also like failing to minister to him. People are dying, both physically and spiritually, and in a very real sense their lives are in your hands. Please don't leave this people group unreached.

RESOURCES

Because websites are constantly changing, it's possible that by the time you read this list, some of the sites may have moved, or the information may no longer correspond to the principles in this book. I believe, however, that the following resources are a good place to start when looking for information and assistance in transitioning to a healthier lifestyle. This is by no means a comprehensive list. Many of the resources listed here will lead to others, which I hope will also be useful.

I believe that the products sold by the suppliers and vendors listed here are good alternatives to those traditionally found on store shelves, but I can't guarantee that every product sold is a good choice, either in general or for any particular buyer. It's always a good idea to test any new product for personal tolerability. This is especially true of building and renovation materials, which aren't easily removed. All buyers need to learn to read ingredients and to be well-informed consumers, but no one needs to feel that they are in this journey alone. There are plenty of people tuning into these issues and lots of company on this road to a healthier future.

Christian Health-Related Ministries

Aroma of Christ Ministry
A Christian ministry to the chemically sensitive
https://www.facebook.com/Aroma-of-Christ-Ministry-315476038471691/

Chronic Joy
A chronic illness ministry
https://chronic-joy.org/

Where is God Ministries
WIGM is designed to encourage people with chronic illnesses and educate their family members and friends. Pamphlets on "Why Go Perfume Free to Church?" are available for purchase.
https://whereisgod.net

Christian Chemical Illness Support Groups

Aroma of Christ
Christian prayer and encouragement email group for those with chemical illness and related conditions
https://groups.io/g/AromaofChrist/

Christians with Environmental Illness
Facebook group
https://www.facebook.com/groups/278736898876252/

CMCS-EI: Christians with Invisible Illnesses
Christian email group for those with chemical sensitivities and other invisible illnesses
https://groups.yahoo.com/neo/groups/CMCS-EI/info

Hope in Him
Hope in Him is an interdenominational ministry that sponsors monthly conference calls.
http://hopeinhimministries2013.org/

St. Teresa's Faith Community
Catholic-focused group that celebrates Evening Prayer and Liturgy of the Word by conference call
https://santacatalinaparish.org/parish-ministries/st-teresas-faith-community/

Church-Related Articles and Informational Pages

Anabaptist Disabilities Network
Multiple Chemical Sensitivity information page
http://www.adnetonline.org/Resources/DisabilityTopics/Hidden-disabilities/Pages/MCS-Tips.aspx

Are You Allergic to Your Church?
Short article from *Hopekeepers* magazine
http://www.restministries.org/hk_mag/09_10_2004/allergic.htm

Chemicals and Christians
The website and blog associated with this book
chemicalsandchristians.com

The CIA Campaign: A Campaign for Cleaner Indoor Air
Printable letter on fragrance and air quality issues addressed to church staff
Links to pamphlets, brochures, flyers, and other resources
https://cleanerindoorair.org/campaigns/fragrance-free-church/

How Accessible is Your Church?
Church accessibility review from The Christian Council on Persons with Disabilities
Covers many disabilities and includes a section on environmental friendliness
http://www.restministries.org/hopekeepers/is-your-church-accessible.pdf

Multiple Chemical Sensitivity Accessibility for United Methodist Churches
Information on MCS taken from *Accessibility Audit for Churches, a United Methodist Resource Book about Accessibility*
http://www.wtv-zone.com/infchoice/mcs/access.html

CHRISTIAN TEACHING AND BIBLE STUDY TOOLS

Back to the Bible
Bible studies, quizzes, and podcast archives
http://www.backtothebible.org/

Bible Gateway
Online Bible with many versions and reading plans
http://www.biblegateway.com/

Bible Hub
Commentaries, Bible studies, and more
https://biblehub.com/

Bible Study Tools
Bibles, reference works, articles, reading plans, and other resources
http://www.biblestudytools.com/

Oneplace
Links to hundreds of Christian radio and online ministries
http://www.oneplace.com/

GENERAL CHEMICAL ILLNESS AND TOXIN AWARENESS RESOURCES

American Academy of Environmental Medicine
Enables patients to search for doctors familiar with chemical illness
http://www.aaemonline.org/

Chemical Injury Information Network
A support and advocacy organization providing resource materials and referrals to experts
http://ciin.org/

The Chemical Sensitivity Foundation

The goal of the organization is to raise public awareness of MCS. Visitors to the site can watch a video discussing the issue.
http://chemicalsensitivityfoundation.org/

The CIA Campaign: A Campaign for Cleaner Air

Advocacy site addressing fragrance and chemical dangers
http://cleanerindoorair.org/

Dr. Anne Steinemann

Links to Dr. Steinemann's studies on chemical toxicity issues
http://www.drsteinemann.com/

The EI Wellspring

Practical information for people with MCS and electromagnetic hypersensitivity
http://www.eiwellspring.org/

HEAL – Human Ecology Action League

One of the oldest organizations concerned about the health effects of environmental exposures
http://www.healnatl.org/

Health Risk Navigation, Inc.

Canadian-based site with links to both US and Canadian resources
https://www.hrni.ca

Hoffman TILT Program

Research and a link to the Quick Environmental Exposure and Sensitivity Inventory (QEESI), a screening instrument for chemical sensitivity
https://tiltresearch.org/

Planet Thrive

An online community for those "ready to kick convention to the curb and reclaim responsibility for their health"
http://planetthrive.com/

Safer Chemicals: Healthy Families

A coalition of 450 organizations and businesses working to remove hazardous chemicals from the marketplace and strengthen regulations.
https://saferchemicals.org/

Seriously Sensitive to Pollution

Comprehensive site with a long list of resources
https://seriouslysensitivetopollution.org/

Think Before You Stink

The site contains information sheets that can be printed and bumper stickers that can be purchased.
http://thinkbeforeyoustink.com/stickers.html

Understanding and Accommodating People with Multiple Chemical Sensitivity in Independent Living

Thorough and compassionate treatment of the needs of the chemically sensitive, including challenges related to healthcare, employment, housing, and psychological losses
http://www.ilru.org/sites/default/files/MCS%20FINAL.PDF

PRODUCT SAFETY INFORMATION

EPA Safer Choice Products

Searchable database of products in many categories
https://www.epa.gov/saferchoice/products

The Environmental Working Group's Guide to Healthy Cleaning

Evaluates and rates the safety of more than 2500 cleaning products
https://www.ewg.org/guides/cleaners

Healthy Stuff

Evaluates the safety of products in many categories, including children's products, pets, cars, and apparel
http://www.healthystuff.org/

Skin Deep: Cosmetic Safety Database
A searchable safety guide to cosmetics and personal care products
https://www.ewg.org/skindeep/

Healthy Building and Renovation

Books

The Healthy House: How to Buy One, How to Cure a Sick One, How to Build One. Fourth Edition, John Bower, Healthy House Institute, Bloomington, IN, 2000

Prescriptions for a Healthy House: A Practical Guide for Architects, Builders, and Homeowners. Paula Baker-Laporte, AIA, Erica Elliott, MD, and John Banta, New Society Publishers, 2001

Online Resources

Considerations for Safer Construction and Renovation
Article by an architect, first published in the *Human Ecologist*
http://www.environmentalhealth.ca/w9394safer.html

Ecology House Property Management and Design Criteria
Descriptions of building materials and methods used in the construction of an environmentally safer housing development
http://www.tikvah.com/cc/eh/evalpt2.html

Heating and Cooling Options for the Environmentally Sensitive
Discussion of gas, electric, hydronic, and passive solar systems
http://eiwellspring.org/HeatingAndCooling.htm

Indoor Air Quality Guide: Best Practices for Design, Construction, and Commissioning
A guide designed for architects, engineers, contractors, and others concerned with air quality in new buildings
https://www.ashrae.org/technical-resources/bookstore/indoor-air-quality-guide

My Chemical-Free House
A guide to building a chemical- and mold-free home
https://www.mychemicalfreehouse.net/

Recommended Architectural Features for Multi-Family Housing to Better Accommodate Chemical and Electrical Sensitivities
Short list of health-related factors to consider in multi-family dwellings
http://ehnca.org/www/ehnlinx/archism.htm

Safer Building Materials for People Who Can't Tolerate Many Commonly Used Chemicals
Article originally published in *Ecological News*
http://cybercilnew.tripod.com/library/building.html

Suppliers

AFM Safecoat
Providers of safer stains, paints, sealers, adhesives, and cleaners, including sealers specifically designed to seal in toxins
http://www.afmsafecoat.com/

E. L. Foust
Providers of air and water filters as well as other healthier home building and improvement products
http://www.foustco.com/

Green Building Supply
Products include cleaners, finishes, countertops, flooring, and environmental testing kits
http://www.greenbuildingsupply.com

The Green Design Center
Large site with many diverse products
https://www.thegreendesigncenter.com/

Nirvana Safe Haven
Focus on beds and bedding, air and water purifiers, and fume and odor control solutions
http://www.nontoxic.com/

Safer Housing

Barrhaven Non-Profit Housing, Inc.
Seven units designed for the environmentally sensitive
http://www.barrhavenunited.org/non_profit_housing.php

EI Safe Housing
Large Facebook group focused on housing issues
https://www.facebook.com/groups/150413784999257/

Ecology House
Eleven-unit low-income housing for the chemically sensitive
http://www.tikvah.com/cc/eh/

MCS/EI Roommate Finder
Facebook group designed to help toxic illness sufferers find shared housing situations
https://www.facebook.com/groups/MCSroommatefinder/

MCS Safe Shelter USA
Email support group with searchable database of homes for sale or rent and roommates wanted
https://groups.yahoo.com/neo/groups/mcssafeshelterusa/info

ReShelter
Charitable corporation founded to address the urgent need for housing alternatives for people with toxic illness
http://reshelter.org/

Nontoxic Cleaning

Books

Clean and Green: The Complete Guide to Non-Toxic and Environmentally Safe Housekeeping, Annie Berthold–Bond, Ceres Press, Woodstock, NY, 1994

Less Toxic Alternatives, Carolyn Gorman, Optimum Publishing, 2002

Nontoxic, Natural, and Earthwise, Debra Lynn Dadd, Tarcher, 1990

Websites

An internet search will bring up many pages of nontoxic cleaning recipes and tips. Remember the cautions in chapter 3.

Eartheasy
http://eartheasy.com/live_nontoxic_solutions.htm

Wellness Mama
https://wellnessmama.com/6244/natural-cleaning/

Lawn Care and Pest Management

Information

The Best Control
Download a free book entitled "The Bug Stops Here"
http://www.thebestcontrol.com/sitemap.htm

Beyond Pesticides
Information on dealing with a variety of common pests
https://www.beyondpesticides.org/resources/managesafe/choose-a-pest

Products

Biocontrol Network
Insect, bird, rodent, and other pest control; lawn, tree, water, and soil care and testing
http://biconet.com/

Gardens Alive
Lawn, soil, and plant care; insect and animal control
http://www.gardensalive.com

Natural Lawn
Fertilizer, grass seed, insect, rodent, and weed control
http://www.naturalawn.com/CoproductForSale.aspx

Planet Natural
Gardening and pest control products
https://www.planetnatural.com/product-category/natural-pest-control/

Services

Some traditional lawn-service companies have organic options, which are obviously better choices than what's usually offered. However, be aware that when you support those companies you may face issues of cross-contamination, and your money also indirectly supports pesticide use. There's a lack of nationwide organic lawn care services in the United States, but local options seem to be becoming more plentiful. An internet search for "nontoxic lawn care" and the name of your city will sometimes give you a helpful result or two.

Canadians Against Pesticides:
Organic Lawn/Garden Care Services and Sites
List of organic lawn care services in Canada
http://www.caps.20m.com/landscape.htm

Natural Lawn of America
Environmentally friendly approach to lawn care available in many states
Franchise opportunities available
http://www.naturalawn.com/

Personal Care Products

NEEDS
Personal care, environmental equipment, clothing, pet care, and other safer products
http://www.needs.com/

Vitacost
Personal care and beauty products, vitamins, food, and more
https://www.vitacost.com/

Travel

Green Vacation Hub
Lists "green" accommodations from around the globe.
https://www.greenvacationhub.com/index.php

ReShelter Safer Travel
Contains a list of safer lodging options for travelers. Follow the "Safer Travel" link from the ReShelter home page.
http://reshelter.org/

Workplace Accommodation

Job Accommodation Network
Information on MCS for employers, including an informational PowerPoint presentation
https://askjan.org/disabilities/Multiple-Chemical-Sensitivity.cfm

Scent-Free Policy for the Workplace
Fact sheet from the Canadian Centre for Occupational Health and Safety
https://www.ccohs.ca/oshanswers/hsprograms/scent_free.html

HEALTHCARE

The CIA Campaign: A Campaign for Cleaner Indoor Air
Printable letter on fragrance and air quality issues addressed to medical providers
https://cleanerindoorair.org/campaigns/fragrance-free-medical/

Healthcare Without Harm
International coalition of hospitals, healthcare systems, medical professionals, and others working to implement healthy alternatives to common healthcare practices
http://www.noharm.org

Hospital protocols
A list of sites linking to hospital protocols for chemically sensitive patients
https://seriouslysensitivetopollution.org/2013/02/17/
hospital-protocols-for-people-with-mcses/

Massachusetts Nurses Association
Position paper on cleaning chemicals in healthcare settings
https://www.massnurses.org/nursing-resources/position-statements/
env-cleaning-chem

Tips for First Responders
Includes a section on assisting those with MCS
http://cdd.unm.edu/dhpd/pdfs/FifthEditionTipsSheet.pdf

Women's College Hospital
Fragrance-free policy
https://www.womenscollegehospital.ca/news-and-publications/connect/
july-8,-2019/wch-is-a-fragrance-free-environment

SAFER SCHOOLS

Healthy Schools Network
National environmental health organization focused on ensuring every child has a healthy learning environment
http://www.healthyschools.org/

IAQ Tools for Schools
Resources for schools from the US Environmental Protection Agency
http://www.epa.gov/iaq/schools/

Nontoxic Pest Management Program for Schools
Description of a nontoxic program currently available to any school district
http://www.getipm.com/schools/ipm-program.htm

DISCUSSION QUESTIONS

CHAPTER ONE

To your knowledge, have you ever had physical symptoms from exposure to chemicals in your environment?

Do you think it's possible that any unexplained condition that you now or have previously experienced could have a chemical connection?

Read 1 Corinthians 6:19–20. How do those verses relate to decisions about what we put in and on our bodies?

Why do you think our society isn't more aware of the problem of chemical illness or of the toxicity of common products?

Why do you think there are so many synthetic chemicals in our environment?

Whose responsibility do you think it is to protect people from toxic exposures?

Were you surprised at the number of people who say they are unusually sensitive to everyday chemicals? Why or why not? Do you know people who fall into that category?

CHAPTER TWO

Have you ever had a medical condition that doctors couldn't explain?

Do you think people tend to make judgments about those who are ill when the diagnosis isn't clear? Have you ever been judged wrongly? How did it feel?

What would be a Christlike response to someone suffering from a medical condition who can find no answers?

Is it important to know why someone is ill before caring for them?

Chapter Three

Read Leviticus 14:36–45. Does this passage shed light on whether or not God cares about toxins in our homes?

Deuteronomy 22:8 is another Scripture that speaks about the responsibility of making a home safe. Do you think the principle in the verse also applies to toxins in the home environment?

How many fragranced products do you use on a daily basis? Have you ever stopped to count?

Have you ever tried cleaning with natural products such as baking soda or vinegar? Why or why not?

Are there changes you think you should make to your home? If so, where and when will you begin?

Chapter Four

Have you ever had a time when something like a broken bone or a similar condition prevented you from entering a public place? Were you able to work around the problem? If so, how? Did you need help from others?

Read Matthew 7:12. What does the Bible say is "the essence of all that is taught in the law and the prophets?" Does that verse pertain to protecting others from the effects of harmful chemicals?

What does 1 John 4:20–21 say about loving God and loving each other?

What is your first thought when you see someone wearing a mask?

Do you think people should attend church even when doing so makes them sick?

Read Romans 10:14. Does this verse apply to making churches accessible to all who wish to enter? What are the consequences when people can't safely attend?

Do you have some control over the air quality in a public place such as a school, an office, or a church? How can you make it a healthier environment?

Chapter Five

Do you believe God generally wants us to seek medical treatment when we are ill? Why or why not?

In 2 Kings 5:1–14, a man named Naaman sought healing, but he almost missed it because it didn't come the way he thought it would. Do you think sick people today sometimes fall into the same trap? Have you ever almost missed God's provision for you because it came in a way you weren't expecting?

Have costs or other prohibitions ever prevented you from pursuing medical treatment?

Have you ever given or received a health-related gift?

What criteria do you think should be used when deciding on medical treatments to pursue?

Why do you think Jesus healed in so many different ways?

Chapter Six

Have you ever had difficulty meeting your basic needs? How did you get around the problem?

Do you make assumptions about homeless people? If so, what do you assume?

How can you help toxic illness sufferers hold onto hope?

How long do you think people should continue to pray for those with chronic medical needs? When should names be removed from prayer lists?

First Corinthians 12:26–27 speaks of the body of Christ. If the whole body suffers because one part does, how do you think that "body parts" cut off because of MCS may impact the body of Christ?

Chapter Seven

First Samuel 1:9–14 tells the story of Hannah who was praying so intensely the priest thought she was drunk. Have you ever been misjudged? Have you misjudged others? Do you think wrong assumptions are often made about the chronically ill?

Do you think you've ever been viewed as a problem rather than as a person? How did it make you feel?

What is your interpretation of Isaiah 53:5? Do you think that earthly physical healing has been promised to all who follow Christ? Why or why not?

What is your understanding of the relationship between sin and suffering?

Chapter Eight

Read James 2:14–17 and discuss the relationship between belief and action.

Have you seen or heard reports painting MCS as a psychosomatic condition or labeling sufferers in a negative way? Is there anything you can do to counteract those messages?

What does 1 Timothy 6:10 note is a root of all kinds of evil? How do you think the verse might relate to the struggles that the chemically sensitive face?

Read Isaiah 1:17. Do you think toxic illness sufferers might fall into the category of "the oppressed"?

Chapter Nine

Why do you think God asked Job to pray for his friends? Do you think it was hard for Job?

1 Thessalonians 5:18 tells us to be thankful in all things. What do you think that means?

In Philippians 4:19, we are promised that God will meet all of our needs. What is your definition of a need?

In Genesis 16:13, Hagar described the Lord as El-Roi, "The God who sees me." What do you think she meant by that? Which of God's names and attributes currently speaks most deeply to you?

Chapter Ten

Is there something you could do to join forces with those helping to raise awareness of chemical sensitivity and of toxins in the environment? Do you feel led to do it?

Have you ever seen a sign or otherwise been asked to attend an event fragrance-free? Do you think that's becoming more common? Are you in a position to help declare a club, a Bible study, or another group a fragrance-free gathering and to reduce the use of other toxins?

What does Galatians 6:9 urge us not to do?

Do you have hope that the air we share will be healthier for future generations? Will you be part of the change?

CHURCH CHECKLIST

There are many areas to consider when attempting to make a church or other building healthier for all and accessible for those with chemical sensitivities. Because of the cumulative nature of toxic exposures, every positive change matters, no matter how small. I urge people not to get overwhelmed by the list of possible changes, but to simply take a step, then take another. Keeping the body of Christ as healthy as possible and making churches accessible to all is worth the effort. The stakes for inaction are high, and they may have eternal consequences.

Questions to Consider

- Is the church cleaned with nontoxic, fragrance-free products? This should be an easy change to make and one that can greatly increase the safety of the air and the health of those who breathe it.

- Are products that the church provides for members' use also nontoxic and fragrance-free? This category may include items such as soaps in the bathrooms or dishwashing products in the kitchen.

- Are there any "air fresheners" of any type (spray, mist, solid, gel, etc.) used in the building? They should be removed.

- How does the church deal with the issue of bugs? Are nontoxic pest-control methods used when necessary?

- How is the lawn maintained? Are safe products chosen?

- Is the church ventilated well and is there provision for adequate air exchange? Are ventilation fans installed? Do windows open?

- How is the building heated and cooled? Is there the possibility for gas, oil, or combustion by-products to affect indoor air? Is there a gas stove in the kitchen that may cause problems for some people?

- When the building is renovated or remodeled, are products and projects chosen with human health in mind? Are low-toxicity paints and sealers selected? Are inert building and flooring materials used?

- Are church members educated about toxicity considerations? Are they asked to refrain from wearing fragranced products in the church environment? Are there notices in the bulletin or on the church website addressing the issue?

- Is provision made for church members who are unable to attend? Are they able to participate in the life of the church through webcasts, audio or video calls, or in other ways?

- Is there at least one Christian church in the area that the chemically sensitive can attend? If not (or even if so), would your church consider building a chemical "safe room" to meet the need?

When Jesus walked the earth in human form, he opened the eyes of many who were blind. I believe that God wants to do the same today. I believe he wants us to see the unintended effects of products we use and to see the almost invisible and largely unreached people group of the chemically sensitive. I pray that God will open our eyes and that we will have the determination and courage to act on what we see.

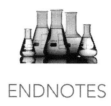

ENDNOTES

Chapter One Notes

1. Pamela Reed Gibson, Amy Nicole-Marie Elms, and Lisa Ann Ruding, "Perceived Treatment Efficacy for Conventional and Alternative Therapies Reported by Persons with Multiple Chemical Sensitivity," *Environmental Health Perspectives* 111, no. 2 (2003): 1498–1504, http://www.ncbi.nlm.nih.gov/pmc/articles/PMC1241653/.

2. Claudia S. Miller, "If You Throw a Magnet in a Computer . . . It TILTs," http://new.drclaudiamiller.com/blog/146-if-you-throw-a-magnet-in-a-computer-it-tilts.

3. Grace Ziem, "Learning about Chemical Injury with Dr. Grace Ziem," previously found at http://www.chemicalinjury.net/videosandmedia.htm.

4. G. Ziem, personal communication, November 13, 2012.

5. National Institute on Drug Abuse, "What Are the Short- and Long-Term Effects of Inhalant Use?" (July 2012): https://www.drugabuse.gov/publications/research-reports/inhalants/what-are-short-long-term-effects-inhalant-use.

6. G. Ziem, personal communication, November 13, 2012.

7. G. Ziem, personal communication, March 15, 2013.

8   Dr. Gerald H. Ross, MD, "Response to Errors Prevalent in the Understanding of Environmental Illness," May 2000, http://www.environmentalhealth.ca/Ross2000.html.

9   Robert W. Haleya, Scott Billecke and Bert N. La Du, "Association of Low PON1 Type Q (Type A) Arylesterase Activity with Neurologic Symptom Complexes in Gulf War Veterans," *Toxicology and Applied Pharmacology* 157, no. 3 (1999): 227–233, http://www.sciencedirect.com/science/article/pii/S0041008X99987033.

10   G. McKeown-Eyssen et al., "Case-Control Study of Genotypes in Multiple Chemical Sensitivity: CYP2D6, NAT1, NAT2, PON1, PON2 and MTHFR," *International Journal of Epidemiology* 33, no. 5 (2004): 971–978, https://www.ncbi.nlm.nih.gov/pubmed/15256524.

11   William J. Meggs, "Hypothesis for Induction and Propagation of Chemical Sensitivity Based on Biopsy Studies," *Environmental Health Perspectives,* 105, suppl. 2 (2004), 473–478, http://www.jstor.org/discover/10.2307/3433355?uid=2&uid=4&sid=21101644233407.

12   Ross, "Response."

13   Ross, "Response."

14   John Molot, M.D., *12,000 Canaries Can't Be Wrong* (Toronto: ECW Press, 2014), 106.

15   Molot, *Canaries*, 104.

16   Diana Crumpler, "Multiple Chemical Sensitivity (MCS) and Electromagnetic Hypersensitivity (EHS): An Introduction to Environmental Illness," *COJ Nursing and Healthcare* (January 22, 2018): https://crimsonpublishers.com/cojnh/fulltext/COJNH.000516.php.

17   Beatrice Alexandra Golomb, "Acetylcholinesterase Inhibitors and Gulf War Illnesses," *Proceedings of the National Academy of Sciences of the United States of America* 105, no. 11 (2008): 4295–4300, http://www.ncbi.nlm.nih.gov/pmc/articles/PMC2393741/.

18 *The Sydney Morning Herald*, "Gulf War Syndrome Frmly Linked to Chemical Exposure" (March 11, 2008): https://www.smh.com.au/world/gulf-war-syndrome-firmly-linked-to-chemical-exposure-20080311-1ymv.html.

19 Eric Schlosser, "Why McDonald's Fries Taste So Good," from *Fast Food Nation* (Houghton-Mifflin, 2001), printed in *The Atlantic Monthly* (January 2001): https://rense.com/general7/whyy.htm.

20 Lynn Lawson, *Staying Well in a Toxic World* (Chicago: Noble Press, 1993), 35.

21 Dr. Mark Donohoe, *Killing Us Softly* (Internet Creative Commons release, 2008), 8, https://static1.squarespace.com/static/54059cd8e4b09fa759f4c83f/t/5416a202e4b00f3a4f0de025/1410769410474/Killing+Us+Softly+1.3.pdf.

22 Nicholas A. Ashford and Claudia S. Miller, *Chemical Exposures: Low Levels and High Stakes* (New York: Van Nostrand Reinhold, 1991), 31.

23 Marla Cone, "Products Derived from Natural, Nontoxic Ingredients—Once Seen as Fringe—Are Now Mainstream," *Los Angeles Times* (September 14, 2008): http://www.latimes.com/local/la-me-greenchem14-2008sep14-story.html.

24 Mike Adams, "Red Alert for Humanity: Chemical Damage can be Inherited by Offspring through Unlimited Generations," *Natural News* (May 24, 2012): http://www.naturalnews.com/035965_epigenetics_inheritance_synthetic_chemicals.html.

25 World Health Organization, "Occupational Risks and Children's Health" (updated December 2009): http://www.who.int/ceh/capacity/occupational.pdf.

26 I. R. Bell et al., "Self-Reported Chemical Sensitivity and Wartime Chemical Exposures in Gulf War Veterans with and without Decreased Global Health Ratings," *Military Medicine* 163 (1998): 725–732, http://www.ncbi.nlm.nih.gov/pubmed/9819530.

27 William J. Meggs et al., "Prevalence and Nature of Allergy and Chemical Sensitivity in a General Population," *Archives of Environmental Health* 51, no. 4 (1996): 275–282, https://www.tandfonline.com/doi/abs/10.1080/00039896.1996.9936026.

28 R. E. Voorhees, "Memorandum from New Mexico Deputy State Epidemiologist to Joe Thompson, Special Counsel, Office of the Governor," March 13,1998.

29 Richard Kreutzer, Raymond R. Neutra and Nan Lashuay, "Prevalence of People Reporting Sensitivities to Chemicals in a Population-Based Survey," *American Journal of Epidemiology*, 150, no. 1 (1999): 1–12, http://aje.oxfordjournals.org/cgi/reprint/150/1/1.

30 Stanley M. Caress and Anne C. Steinemann, "The National Prevalence of Chemical Hypersensitivity, the Medical Diagnosis of Multiple Chemical Sensitivities, and Potential Overlaps with Asthma," *Townsend Letter for Doctors and Patients* (2005): http://www.tandfonline.com/doi/abs/10.3200/AEOH.58.6.300-305.

31 Anne Steinemann, PhD, "National Prevalence and Effects of Multiple Chemical Sensitivities," *Journal of Occupational and Environmental Medicine*, 60, no. 3 (2018) https://journals.lww.com/joem/Fulltext/2018/03000/National_Prevalence_and_Effects_of_Multiple.17.aspx.

32 Steinemann, "National Prevalence."

33 Alison Johnson, *Casualties of Progress: Personal Histories from the Chemically Sensitive* (Brunswick, ME: MCS Information Exchange), 261.

34 Howard M. Kipen, MD et al., "Measuring Chemical Sensitivity Prevalence: A Questionnaire for Population Studies," *American Journal of Public Health* 85, no. 4 (1995): 574–577, http://ajph.aphapublications.org/doi/pdf/10.2105/AJPH.85.4.574.

35 David A. Katerndahl, MD, MA et al., "Chemical Intolerance in Primary Care Settings: Prevalence, Comorbidity, and Outcomes,"

Annals of Family Medicine 10, no. 4 (2012): 357–365, http://annfammed.org/content/10/4/357.

36   Claudia S. Miller and Nicholas A. Ashford, *Multiple Chemical Sensitivities: Addendum to Biological Markers in Immunotoxicology* (National Academies Press, 1992), p. 60.

37   Lawson, *Staying Well*, 36.

38   G. Ziem, personal communication, November 13, 2012.

39   Robert D. Brook et al., "Particulate Matter Air Pollution and Cardiovascular Disease," *Circulation* 121 (2010): 2331–2378, http://circ.ahajournals.org/content/121/21/2331.full.pdf.

40   Matthew 22:39.

41   U.S. Environmental Protection Agency, Toxicity and Exposure Assessment for Children's Health (TEACH), Chemical Summaries, https://archive.epa.gov/region5/teach/web/html/teachsummaries.html.

42   "Absolute Astronomy," Encyclopedia, Zyklon B, http://www.absoluteastronomy.com/topics/Zyklon_B.

43   Heather Hamlin, "Pesticides Blamed for Some Childhood Brain Cancers," *Environmental Health News*, April 7, 2009, https://www.organicconsumers.org/scientific/pesticides-blamed-some-childhood-brain-cancers.

44   Elizabeth Grossman, "Chemicals May Play Role in Rise in Obesity," *Special to The Washington Post* (March 12, 2007): http://www.mdpestnet.org/chemicals-may-play-role-in-rise-in-obesity/.

45   Ashford and Miller, *Chemical Exposures*, 170–177.

46   Marla Cone, "Scientists Find 'Baffling' Link between Autism and Vinyl Flooring," *Environmental Health News* (March 31, 2009): https://www.scientificamerican.com/article/link-between-autism-and-vinyl/.

47   Francesca Lyman, "What the Nose Knows: Think Twice before Buying a Loved One Perfume, Cologne" (February 12,

2003): http://www.nbcnews.com/id/3076635/ns/health-your_environment/t/what-nose-knows/#.W7u_yWhKg2w.

48 Brandy E. Fisher, "Scents & Sensitivity," *Environmental Health Perspectives* 106, no. 12 (1998): 594–599, http://www.herc.org/news/perfume/EHPscents.htm.

49 "Chemical Sensitivities and Perfume," *Medical News Today* (June 19, 2004): http://www.medicalnewstoday.com/articles/9682.php.

50 Tracy Fernandez Rysavy, "Heal Your Home: The Case for Precaution," *Green American*, Spring 2008, https://www.greenamerica.org/heal-your-home-case-precaution.

51 "Lautenberg, Solis, Waxman Introduce Legislation to Protect Americans from Hazardous Chemicals in Consumer Products," *Medical News Today* (May 21, 2008): http://www.medicalnewstoday.com/articles/108253.php.

52 David Biello, "Are Some Chemicals More Dangerous at Low Dosage?" *Scientific American* (April 3, 2009): https://blogs.scientificamerican.com/news-blog/are-some-chemicals-more-dangerous-a-2009-04-03/.

53 Al Meyerhoff, "Chemicals: Our Champions, Our Killers," *Los Angeles Times* (December 28, 2008): http://www.latimes.com/la-oe-meyerhoff28-2008dec28-story.html.

54 Safer Chemicals, Healthy Families, "An Abbreviated Guide to the Frank R. Lautenberg Chemical Safety for the 21st Century Act," https://saferchemicals.org/public-policy/an-abbreviated-guide.

55 Lawson, *Staying Well*, 365.

56 David Biello, "Are Some Chemicals More Dangerous at Low Dosage?" *Scientific American*, April 3, 2009, https://blogs.scientificamerican.com/news-blog/are-some-chemicals-more-dangerous-a-2009-04-03/.

57 David Biello, "Mixing it Up: Harmless Levels of Chemicals Prove Toxic Together," *Scientific American* (May 2006): https://www.scientificamerican.com/article/mixing-it-up/.

58   Donohoe, *Killing Us,* 38.

59   Lawson, *Staying Well*, 88.

60   "No More Toxic Tub: Getting Contaminants Out of Children's Bath & Personal Care Products," The Campaign for Safe Cosmetics (March 12, 2009): http://www.safecosmetics.org/wp-content/uploads/2016/12/NoMoreToxicTub_Report_Mar09.pdf.

61   Lorraine Smith, *Heal Environmental Illness and Reclaim Your Life* (Chelmsford, MA: Diveena Publications, 2000), 27.

Chapter Two Notes

62   Johnson, *Casualties*, 128.

63   Elizabeth Cohen, "Has Your Illness Been Misdiagnosed?" CNN Health, http://www.cnn.com/2007/HEALTH/09/19/ep.misdiagnoses/index.html.

64   Stephen G. Pelletier, "Experts See Growing Importance of Adding Environmental Health Content to Medical School Curricula," AAMC News (September 26, 2016): https://news.aamc.org/medical-education/article/experts-importance-environmental-health-content/.

65   Gibson, "Treatment Efficacy,"1498–1504, http://www.ncbi.nlm.nih.gov/pmc/articles/PMC1241653/.

66   "The Usual Suspect," *Newsweek* (February 14, 2009): http://www.newsweek.com/id/184155.

67   Diana Crumpler, "Multiple Chemical Sensitivity (MCS) and Electromagnetic Hypersensitivity (EHS): An Introduction to Environmental Illness," *COJ Nursing and Healthcare* (January 22, 2018): https://crimsonpublishers.com/cojnh/fulltext/COJNH.000516.php.

68   Donohoe, *Killing Us*, 26–27.

69   Pamela Reed Gibson, PhD, *Multiple Chemical Sensitivity: A Survival Guide* (Oakland, CA: New Harbinger Publications, 2000), 156.

70   Johnson, *Casualties*, 4.

71   Johnson, *Casualties*, 2.

72   Johnson, *Casualties*, 5.

73   Johnson, *Casualties*, 124.

74   Jim Andrews, *Polishing God's Monuments: Pillars of Hope for Punishing Times* (Wapwallopen, Penn: Shepherd Press, 2007), 79.

75   Johnson, *Casualties*, 186.

76   Christa and Steve Upton, *MCS: Banished from the Human Race* (Black Hills Picture Books, 2017), 43.

77   Johnson, *Casualties*, 127.

78   Johnson, *Casualties*, 12.

79   Flora Preston, *Convenient, "Safe" and Deadly: The True Costs of Our Chemical Lifestyle* (Lanark, Ontario, Health Risk Navigation, Inc., 2006), 51.

80   Gibson, "Treatment Efficacy," 1498–1504, http://www.ncbi.nlm.nih.gov/pmc/articles/PMC1241653/.

81   Johnson, *Casualties*, 60.

82   Angela Cummings, "Sick House Syndrome: 3 Strategies for a home that may be making you sick," RUAN (June 21, 2017): https://www.nontoxicliving.tips/blog/sick-house-syndrome-3-strategies-for-a-home-that-may-be-making-you-sick.

Chapter Three Notes

83   1 Corinthians 6:19.

84   Lawson, *Staying Well*, 278.

85   Julia Kendall, "Fabric Softeners = Health Risks (from Dryer
      Exhaust and Treated Fabrics)," http://www.herc.org/news/perfume/
      fabric.htm.

86   B. Williams, "The Toxic Danger of Fabric Softener and Dryer
      Sheets,"http://ezinearticles.com/?The-Toxic-Danger-of-Fabric-
      Softener-and-Dryer-Sheets&id=16953.

87   Leviticus 14:33–45.

88   Lawson, *Staying Well*, 234.

89   William A. Rutala, PhD, et al., "Bacterial Contamination of
      Keyboards: Efficacy and Functional Impact of Disinfectants,"
      Infection Control and Hospital Epidemiology 27, no. 4 (2006):
      372–377, https://www.ncbi.nlm.nih.gov/pubmed/16622815.

90   Andrea E Berendt et al., "Three Swipes and You're Out: How
      Many Swipes are Needed to Decontaminate Plastic with
      Disposable Wipes?" *American Journal of Infection Control* 39, issue
      5 (2011): 442–443, https://www.ajicjournal.org/article/S0196-
      6553(10)00935-1/abstract.

91   Judy Stouffer, "Vinegar and Hydrogen Peroxide as Disinfectants,
      "*Science News* 154, no. 6 (1998): 83–85.

92   Annie Berthold-Bond, *Clean and Green* (Woodstock, NY: Ceres
      Press, 1990), Introduction.

93   Environmental Working Group, "EWG's Guide to Healthy
      Cleaning," https://www.ewg.org/guides/categories/2-AllPurpose.

94   Lawson, *Staying Well*, 181.

95   J. Walter Veirs, "Capitol Concerns," *Indoor Pollution Law Report 3*,
      September 1988.

96   Gibson, *Survival Guide*, 50.

97   Robert Uhlig, "Carpets Are Piled High with Toxic Pollutants,"
      Telegraph (May 10, 2001): https://www.telegraph.co.uk/news/
      uknews/1328875/Carpets-are-piled-high-with-toxic-pollutants.
      html.

98   Jane Kay, "Study Says Household Dust Holds Dangerous
        Chemicals: Homes in Seven States Tested for Residues of Consumer
        Goods," *San Francisco Chronicle* (March 23, 2005): http://articles.
        sfgate.com/2005-03-23/news/17366619_1_chemicals-dust-test-
        animals.

99   Robert Uhlig, "Carpets Are Piled High With Toxic Pollutants,"
        Telegraph, May 10, 2001, https://www.telegraph.co.uk/news/
        uknews/1328875/Carpets-are-piled-high-with-toxic-pollutants.
        html.

100   Uhlig, "Carpets."

101   Lawson, *Staying Well*, 6.

102   "Ex-Holy Cross Football Coach Dies from Multiple Chemical
        Sensitivity," Catholic News Service, http://www.wtv-zone.com/
        infchoice/mcs/allen.html.

103   Jackie MacMullen, "Crusader's Toughest Fight," Boston Globe
        (September 2003): http://www.wtv-zone.com/infchoice/mcs/news/
        coach4.html.

104   "Formaldehyde—Advice from US EPA," Healthy House Institute,
        http://www.healthyhouseinstitute.com/a-740-Formaldehyde---
        Advice-from-US-EPA.

105   Agency for Toxic Substances and Disease Registry, Medical
        Management Guidelines for Formaldehyde, http://www.atsdr.cdc.
        gov/mmg/mmg.asp?id=216&tid=39.

106   John Bower, *The Healthy House, 4th Edition* (Bloomington, IN: The
        Healthy House Institute, 2001), 114.

107   "Don't Hold Your Breath: Indoor CO2 Exposure and Impaired
        Decision Making," Environmental Health Perspectives 120, no.12
        (December 2012): https://www.ncbi.nlm.nih.gov/pmc/articles/
        PMC3548304/.

108   Bower, *The Healthy House*, 114.

109   Lawson, *Staying Well*, 142.

110 "What are the Pros and Cons of a Heat Pump vs. a Gas Furnace? Air Master Heating and Air. http://www.airmasterheatingandair. com/what-are-the-pros-and-cons-of-a-heat-pump-vs-a-gas-furnace. html.

111 Preston, *Convenient*, 116.

112 Lawson, *Staying Well*, 59.

113 O. R. McCarthy, "The Key to the Sanatoria," *Journal of the Royal Society of Medicine* 94, no. 8 (2001), 413–417. https://www.ncbi. nlm.nih.gov/pmc/articles/PMC1281640/.

114 Lawson, *Staying Well*, 84.

115 John Bower, *Understanding Ventilation* (Bloomington, IN: The Healthy House Institute, 1995), 178.

116 Bower, *Understanding Ventilation*, 57.

Chapter Four Notes

117 *Women and Environments International Journal,* Vol. 62/63, Spring 2004 (as cited in *The Canary Connection* 2010 Issue 1).

118 Anne C. Steinemann et al., "Chemical Emissions from Residential Dryer Vents during Use of Fragranced Laundry Products," *Air Quality, Atmosphere and Health* (2011): http:// safer-world.org/wp-content/uploads/2011/05/Steinemann-et-al.- AQAH-6-2013-151-156-1.pdf.

119 Dina El Shammaa, "Battling Hala Alive After Toxic Pesticide Fumes Killed Siblings," *Gulf News* (April 2, 2010): http://gulfnews. com/news/gulf/uae/general/battling-hala-alive-after-toxic-pesticide- fumes-killed-siblings-1.606723.

120 Johnson, *Casualties*, 157.

121 Gibson, *Survival Guide*, 33.

122   D. J. Ross, H. L. Keynes, and J. C. McDonald, "SWORD '97: Surveillance of Work-Related and Occupational Respiratory Disease in the UK," *Occupational Medicine* 48, no. 8 (1998): 481–485, http://occmed.oxfordjournals.org/content/48/8/481.abstract.

123   Lawson, *Staying Well*, 114.

124   Lawson, *Staying Well*.

125   Lawson, *Staying Well*, 104.

126   Johnson, *Casualties*, 248.

127   John P. Thomas, "The Addictive Power of Toxic Perfumes and Colognes," Health Impact News (June 18, 2014): https://healthimpactnews.com/2014/the-addictive-power-of-toxic-perfumes-and-colognes/.

128   Johnson, 44.

129   Gibson, "Treatment Efficacy," 1498–1504, http://www.ncbi.nlm.nih.gov/pmc/articles/PMC1241653/.

130   Johnson, *Casualties*, 83.

131   "Girl's Illness Traced to 'Toxic' School," *ABC News*, Good Morning America (October 11, 2005): https://abcnews.go.com/GMA/Health/story?id=1202564&page=1.

132   Delen Goldberg, "Bill Before New York State Lawmakers Would Ban Use of Pesticides on School Playing Fields," *The Post-Standard*, Syracuse, NY (April 20, 2010): http://www.syracuse.com/news/index.ssf/2010/04/post_206.html.

133   Preston, *Convenient*, 98–99.

134   Johnson, *Casualties*, 77.

135   Donohoe, *Killing Us*, 27.

136   Donohoe, 42.

137   "The Proustian Effect," Scent Air, http://www.scentairmena.com/proust.html.

138   Revelation 12:9.

139 Jeff Gearhart and Hans Posselt, "Toxic at Any Speed: Chemicals in Cars and the Need for Safe Alternatives," A Report by The Ecology Center, January 2006.

140 Janine Ridings, *Comfort in the Storm* (Enumclaw, WA: Pleasant Word, 2004), 50.

141 Allan Chernoff and Laura Dolan, "Scientists Analyze Blood to Test for Toxic Airplane Air Exposure," CNN (August 16, 2009): http://www.cnn.com/2009/US/08/17/bleed.air.tests/index.html.

142 E. Millqvist and O. Lowhagen, "Placebo-Controlled Challenges with Perfume in Patients with Asthma-Like Symptoms," *Allergy* 51, no. 6 (1996): 434–439, http://onlinelibrary.wiley.com/doi/10.1111/j.1398-9995.1996.tb04644.x/abstract.

143 Lawson, *Staying Well*, 112.

CHAPTER FIVE NOTES

144 Gibson, "Treatment Efficacy,"1498–1504, http://www.ncbi.nlm.nih.gov/pmc/articles/PMC1241653/.

145 Kim Palmer, "MCS History Summary" (2000): http://www.angelfire.com/az/ox/kim-palmer-story.html.

146 Gibson, *Survival Guide*, 111.

147 Gibson, "Treatment Efficacy," 1498–1504, http://www.ncbi.nlm.nih.gov/pmc/articles/PMC1241653/.

148 1 Timothy 5:23.

149 Matthew 14:35–36.

150 John 5:5, 9:6.

151 Matthew 8:16, Mark 1:34.

152 John 9:3.

153 John 9:6.

154 Gibson, *Survival Guide*, 111.

155   "Learning What Works Best: The Nation's Need for Evidence on Comparative Effectiveness in Health Care: An Issue Overview," Institute of Medicine (US) Roundtable on Value & Science-Driven Health Care. National Academies Press (September 2007): https://www.ncbi.nlm.nih.gov/books/NBK64784/.

156   John 8:44, Revelation 12:9.

157   Mark 3:22.

Chapter Six Notes

158   Luke 12:23.

159   Lawson, *Staying Well*, 210.

160   Upton, *MCS*, 31.

161   Upton, 49.

162   Gibson, "Treatment Efficacy," 1498–1504, http://www.ncbi.nlm.nih.gov/pmc/articles/PMC1241653/.

163   Pamela Reed Gibson, Jennifer Cheavens, and Margaret L. Warren, "Chemical Sensitivity/Chemical Injury and Life Disruption," *Women & Therapy 19* (1996): 63–79, https://www.tandfonline.com/doi/abs/10.1300/J015v19n02_06.

164   "Homelessness at Critical Level for Western Massachusetts Chemically Injured," Environmental Health Coalition of Western Mass. (March 11, 2002): http://www.scribd.com/doc/46547075/Environmental-Health-Group-2002-MCS-Housing-Survey.

165   Upton, *MCS*, 27.

166   "Homelessness at Critical Level for Western Massachusetts Chemically Injured," Environmental Health Coalition of Western Mass. (March 11, 2002): http://www.scribd.com/doc/46547075/Environmental-Health-Group-2002-MCS-Housing-Survey.

167   Christina Elwell, "Disabled Woman Still Seeking a Helping Hand," *Venice Gondolier Sun* (November 20, 2005): http://ufdc.ufl.edu/UF00028295/00135.

168   Ecology House, San Rafael, California, http://www.tikvah.com/cc/eh/.

169   Caryl Schonbrun, "The New Homeless," http://www.mcs-international.org/downloads/105_the_new_homeless.pdf.

170   Ridings, *Comfort*, 204.

171   Gibson, *Survival Guide*, 149.

172   Ridings, *Comfort*, 264.

173   Johnson, *Casualties*, 202.

174   Johnson, 146.

175   1 Timothy 5:23.

176   1 Kings 19:4 and Numbers 11:15.

177   Job 1:1.

178   Job 2:.7.

179   1 Peter 1:7.

CHAPTER SEVEN NOTES

180   1 Samuel 1:12–14.

181   Romans 12:15.

182   Psalm 147:3.

183   3 John 1:1–3.

184   John 5:14.

185   John 5:13.

186   Luke 13:2–3.

187   Job 1:12.

188   Job 12:5.

189   Job 22:5.

190   Gibson, "Treatment Efficacy,"1498–1504, http://www.ncbi.nlm. nih.gov/pmc/articles/PMC1241653/.

191   Bible Hub, https://biblehub.com/greek/1112.htm.

192   Psalm 4:4, Ephesians 4:26–27.

193   Kelly Minter, *Ruth: Loss, Love, and Legacy* (Nashville: Lifeway Press, 2009), 41.

Chapter Eight Notes

194   Job 19:2.5.

195   Ann McCampbell, MD, "Multiple Chemical Sensitivities under Siege," *Townsend Letter for Doctors and Patients* (2001): http://www. getipm.com/personal/mcs-campbell.htm.

196   "Homelessness at Critical Level for Western Massachusetts Chemically Injured," Environmental Health Coalition of Western Mass. (March 11, 2002): http://www.scribd.com/doc/46547075/ Environmental-Health-Group-2002-MCS-Housing-Survey.

197   Ashford and Miller, *Chemical Exposures*, 156.

198   Smith, *Heal*, 52.

199   Smith, 54.

200   Smith, 78.

201   Smith, 206.

202   Smith, 174.

203   Johnson, *Casualties*, 60.

CHAPTER NINE NOTES

204   Gregg Easterbrook, "Rx for Life: Gratitude," Beliefnet, http://www. beliefnet.com/Holistic-Living/2000/11/Rx-For-Life-Gratitude. aspx?p=1.

205   Ridings, *Comfort*, 103.

206   Matthew 26:39, *The Message*.

207   Alfred Tennyson, "The Higher Pantheism," *The Holy Grail and Other Poems* (London: Strahan, 1870): https://www. poetryfoundation.org/poems/45323/the-higher-pantheism.

208   Psalm 50:10.

209   1 John 4:8.

210   Hebrews 13:5.

211   Matthew 11:28.

212   Philippians 4:7.

213   Judges 16.

214   Ezekiel 3:24.

215   Posted to the Aroma of Christ email support group, January 15, 2010.

216   Richard Jerome and Margaret Nelson, "Toxic Avenger: Poisoned by Pesticides, A Prisoner in Her Home, Cindy Duehring Wages Global War on Chemicals," *People Magazine* (February 9, 1997): http:// www.wtv-zone.com/infchoice/news/peoples/avenger.html.

217   "Cindy Duehring (USA)," The Right Livelihood Award (1997): https://www.rightlivelihoodaward.org/?s=duehring.

218   "Held Captive in Her Own Home (Part 3)," from *Bismarck Tribune* (November 1997): http://www.wtv-zone.com/infchoice/news/ bismarck/captive3.html.

219   Genesis 1–3.

220   Romans 6:23, Hebrews 9:27.

221   Romans 3:23, 5:12.

222   Isaiah 59:2, John 3:26, Ephesians 2:1.

223   2 Cor. 5:21, 1 Peter 3:18.

224   1 Peter 2:22–24, 1 John 3:5, Romans 6:4–5.

225   John 1:12, John 3:16–18.

Chapter Ten Notes

226   Building Air Quality: A Guide for Building Owners and Facility Managers, US Environmental Protection Agency (December 1991): http://www.cdc.gov/niosh/docs/91-114/pdfs/91-114.pdf.

227   "Chemical Exposures, Fragrance-Free Information," *Massachusetts Nurse Newsletter* (April 2006): http://www.massnurses.org/health-and-safety/articles/chemical-exposures/p/openItem/1346.

228   Pat Seremet, "Spritzed to the Max; To Chemically Sensitive, It Smells like Mean Spirits," *Hartford Courant* (June 1, 2003): http://www.courant.com/news/connecticut/hc-xpm-2003-06-01-0306011889-story.html.

229   "Fragrance-Free Information," Shutesbury, MA, http://www.shutesbury.org/ada_fragrance.

230   Truman Taylor, "Fragrance-Free Shutesbury," *The Providence Journal*, May 4, 2003.

231   Jennifer Steinhauer, "Breath of Fresh Air, Indoors, in Las Vegas," *New York Times* (May 26, 2010): http://www.nytimes.com/2010/05/26/us/26perfume.html.

232   Kate Grenville, *The Case against Fragrance* (Melbourne: The Text Publishing Company, 2017), 152–153.

233   Singer, *Sweet Smell,* http://www.nytimes.com/2008/02/14/fashion/14skin.html?pagewanted=all.

234 "U.S. Home Fragrance Market Glows in 2017." Global Cosmetics Industry (June 26, 2018): https://www.gcimagazine.com/marketstrends/segments/candle/US-Home-Fragrance-Market-Glows-in-2017---486485811.html?utm_source=Most+Read&utm_medium=website&utm_campaign=Most+Read.

235 Everett Jones et al., "School Policies and Practices that Improve Indoor Air Quality," *Journal of School Health* 80, no. 6 (2010): 280–286, http://www.ncbi.nlm.nih.gov/pubmed/20573140.

236 Sample Fragrance-Free School Policy, American Lung Association, http://action.lung.org/site/DocServer/fragrance-free-policy-sample-updated.pdf.

237 Gary L. Glendening, "Westmoreland Elementary Pilots Nontoxic Cleaning," Rock Creek USD 323, Westmoreland Elementary: News, August 19, 2008.

238 Nontoxic Pest Management Program for Schools, The Best Control, http://www.getipm.com/schools/endorsements/fruitport.htm.

239 Delen Goldberg, "Bill Before New York State Lawmakers Would Ban Use of Pesticides on School Playing Fields," *The Post-Standard* (April 20, 2010): http://www.syracuse.com/news/index.ssf/2010/04/post_206.html.

240 Delen Goldberg, "Gov. David Paterson Signs Bill Banning Pesticides on School Playing Fields," *The Post-Standard* (May 18, 2010): http://www.syracuse.com/news/index.ssf/2010/05/gov_david_paterson_signs_bill_1.html.

241 Sara Schilling, "Oasis School in Richland to Close, Leaders Say," *Tri-City Herald*, April 21, 2010.

242 Health Care Without Harm, http://www.noharm.org/.

243 "Chemical Exposures, Fragrance-Free Information," *Massachusetts Nurse Newsletter* (April 2006): http://www.massnurses.org/health-and-safety/articles/chemical-exposures/p/openItem/1346.

244 "Fragrance-Free Policy," Women's College Hospital, https://www. womenscollegehospital.ca/news-and-publications/Connect-2017/ wch-is-a-fragrance-free-environment.

245 Kelly Brewington, "Md. Hospitals, Care Facilities Working to Cut Their Use of Toxic Pesticides," *Baltimore Sun* (October 28, 2008): http://www.beyondpesticides.org/hospitals/media/ BaltimoreSun.10.28.08.inprint.pdf.

246 Wikipedia, Pesticides in Canada. https://en.wikipedia.org/wiki/ Pesticides_in_Canada.

247 Gordy Holt, "Goats Provide Alternative to Chemicals for Weed Control," *Seattle Post-Intelligencer* (August 3, 2005): http://seattlepi. nwsource.com/local/234984_ncenter03.html.

248 Marla Cone, "A Greener Future: Part 1: Products Derived from Natural, Nontoxic Ingredients—Once Seen as Fringe—Are Now Mainstream," *Los Angeles Times* (September 14, 2008): http://www. latimes.com/local/la-me-greenchem14-2008sep14-story.html.

249 "Multiple Chemical Sensitivity," Anabaptist Disabilities Network, http://www.adnetonline.org/Resources/DisabilityTopics/Hidden-disabilities/Pages/MCS-Tips.aspx.

250 "Multiple Chemical Sensitivity Accessibility for United Methodist Churches," from *Accessibility Audit for Churches, A United Methodist Resource Book about Accessibility,* 9–10, http://www.wtv-zone.com/ infchoice/mcs/access.html.

251 "How Accessible Is Your Church?" Christian Council on Persons with Disabilities, http://www.restministries.org/hopekeepers/is-your-church-accessible.pdf.

252 Don Hooser, "Fragrance-Free Rooms, The Risks and Disadvantages of Having to Rely on Them" (January 13, 2002): http://kubik.org/ health/fragrancefree.htm.

253 "Parish Offers Incense-Free Christmas Mass," Associated Press (December 24, 2003): http://www.toxicsinfo.org/personal/ ChristmasMass.htm.

254 Leanne Larmondin, "Scent-Free Parishes in Vogue," *Anglican Journal* (October 1, 2001): https://www.anglicanjournal.com/scent-free-parishes-in-vogue-1332/.

255 "Chemically Sensitive Find Sanctuary in Fragrance-Free Churches," *Huffington Post* (October 26, 2013): https://www.huffingtonpost.com/2013/10/26/chemical-sensitivity-fragrance-church_n_4163785.html.

256 Estelle Taylor, "Barrhaven Project: Safe Houses for the Hypersensitive," *Peace and Environment News*, June 1995.

257 Leah V. Harris, *Jackson Citizen Patriot*, January 24, 2005.

258 Janine Ridings, "Exiled by MCS: A Survivor's Perspective," Poisoned by Malathion, http://www.getipm.com/articles/malathion-reinhardt.htm.

259 "Hazards in the Worship Place," DFW Lighthouse, October 2001 (from an article by Kristin Searfoss in *Presbyterians Today*, May 1999).

Order Information

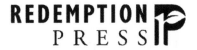

To order additional copies of this book, please visit
www.redemption-press.com.
Also available on Amazon.com and BarnesandNoble.com
Or by calling toll free 1-844-2REDEEM.